AF824493

Stem Cells for Chronic Obstructive Pulmonary Disease (COPD)

ISBN: 978-1-963592-22-1
ISBN: 978-1-963592-23-8
ISBN: 978-1-963592-03-0

Published by Will Bozeman

For more information:
http://www.willbozeman.com

Table of Contents

WILL BOZEMAN

Willbozeman.com
Will@willbozeman.com

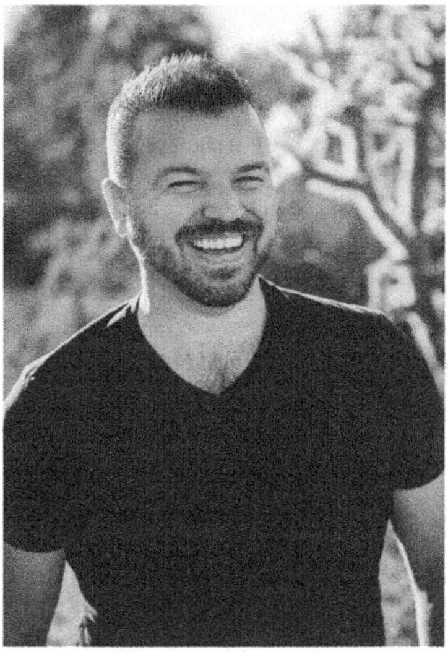

Will is a healthcare executive, innovator, entrepreneur, inventor, and writer with a wide range of experience in the medical field. Will has multiple degrees in a wide range of subjects that give depth to his capability as an entrepreneur and capacity to operate as an innovative healthcare executive. Will has an associate degree in electrical technology, two undergraduate degrees in biotechnology and archaeology, an MBA, and attended medical school in Alabama.

Will took a leave of absence from medical school to open his first biotech lab and serve as the chief science officer, writer, and innovator. Will has founded and launched multiple biotech ventures while serving in a range of positions in that field as chief executive officer, chief science officer, chief medical officer, founder, and innovator. Will has brought multiple biologic products to market for clinical use applications and written many treatment protocols for application of use and helped pioneer the use of regenerative medicine in the medical field.

Prologue

What an exciting age of medicine we live in today!

Stem cells and stem cell applications are already one of the greatest discoveries of modern medicine, and the vast majority of our advanced stem cell medical applications and uses are yet to come.

At the time of writing, there are countless studies on the clinical and medical application of stem cells on musculoskeletal conditions like osteoarthritis and a range of muscle/joint/bone treatments.

Additionally, treatments and research range from very specific disease conditions like specific cancers and congenital diseases, to more general use stem cell treatments for systemic inflammation, anti-aging and longevity, and even for use in aesthetic treatments like high-end facials, skin rejuvenation, and hair regrowth.

Of course, some of the really interesting applications that researchers have their eyes on these days are advancements in nerve tissue regeneration and organ tissue growth and development.

I, for one, am excited for the day when we can simply grow organs for replacement instead of having a transplant list. Also, how about treating a range of chronic illnesses with a simple IV stem cell application on a regular basis using your own stem cells that you own?

I talk about this a lot as the best option for someone considering a stem cell treatment. It's possible now to have your own stem cells collected and have those cells cultured and grown into hundreds of vials of pure stem cells that can be used the rest of your life for anything you need! It's the future of stem cell therapy. I'll explain how all this works later.

There is no shortage of potential applications for use that are coming in the future. However, for the purposes of this book, I want to zero in on what is happening and available right now, what is available to patients in the United States, and what is available at the international stem cell treatment level. There's a lot more available today than you may be aware of!

Most doctors are unfamiliar with all the treatment options available and accessible in the US market today.

My background and history in regenerative medicine

My background in stem cell biotechnology began with my biotech undergraduate degree, where I routinely performed a range of cellular biotech functions, culturing and expanding various cell lines and isolating cellular DNA, and I conducted a range of lab testing procedures to prepare us for the exciting world of cellular biotech.

One of my favorite undergraduate projects that really helped me understand the details of the science of cellular biotechnology was to build a new cell culture lab for our university biotech department.

This project really opened my eyes to how a cell culture lab worked and operated from start to finish. I didn't just learn how to do only specific tasks, like most students; I learned how everything worked, and the how and why behind it. I built the lab that the other students were using to learn, so I had to set it all up the right way for their training, so I had to be one step ahead of the rest of the class to be able to do this.

I learned all about the current state of the industry because I had to build the lab. I had to order and test equipment; determine capabilities and functional uses; troubleshoot lab problems, operations and activity flow of the lab; determine the capabilities of what could be produced in a cell culture lab; and, of course, understand where the industry needed innovation and what was on the horizon.

Most students only got a tiny window into this world, but I was able to stand in front of a huge bay window and see what cellular biotech was all about. This is what really helped me understand the foundation of the world of regenerative medicine and started me down the path of stem cell therapy and regenerative medical applications.

Biotechnology is a notoriously risky field to be in because the people who are often exceptional with the science are not often exceptional with the business and practical applications. Luckily, I snagged my MBA before medical school, so I have a little more understanding of the business of a biotech operation and how to make it succeed.

It doesn't matter how lofty or noble your biotech ambitions are, if you can't pay your bills, you can't do anything to further your efforts … and people don't seem to like working for free. I bring this up because there are a lot of negative impressions regarding medical and business interactions. It's just part of this field. Everyone in the process is educated and requires better than average income, so it's just an expensive field to operate in.

Business and biotech are highly intertwined. Because there are so many variables to account for, biotechnology remains one of the more difficult categories of business to engage in, and yet it continues to attract hundreds and even thousands of new startups and ventures every year.

I believe this is because of the allure of the magnitude of what can be accomplished or what could be developed if your idea or venture succeeds.

The potential upside for success is more enticing than the risk/fear of failure. I've felt this strange dynamic many times. I'm looking at a potentially life-saving therapy and I can immediately convince myself that I would sacrifice my own financial security to get this treatment to market!

I tell you this because this new era of amazing medical therapy is brought to you by innovators and pioneers in this field who often ride the edge of success all the way to the end, good or bad.

Particularly in the world of stem cells, the people I meet are not just thinking of how to start a business or get a good job, they are thinking of how to change the world! The potential for stem cell therapy to revolutionize many categories of medicine is very strong, and this is what drives everyone in this field.

I myself am guilty of diving headfirst into biotech startups because the potential benefits and applications are so exciting that I can't say no. To the surprise of my professors, I started my first lab company, stem cell processing, and storage lab while I was in my biotech undergrad program.

It provided private processing and cryopreservation storage of cord blood and tissue for later stem cell therapies for parents who wanted that protection and assurance for their children.

My professors hadn't seen many students apply what they had learned so quickly in real life. I found myself in real-world conversations with professors over my company and the potential growth and expansion of my startup.

I had conversations with my professors, literally on the side of the classroom, discussing investment and growth options while other students completed their regular course work. I tell you this because my undergrad experience was completely different from that of my peers.

This particular lab operation to process and store cord blood stem cells for parents having children who wanted to save those cells was more than just a business venture; I saw it as a calling, my first real life stem cell operation.

Cord blood stem cells provide a specific type of stem cell that could become valuable to a patient if they develop certain medical conditions down the road, but the only sure fire way to know you have a match available when you need it is to bank it yourself for later. This is exactly what I promote now for adults in the stem cell treatment world, to bank their own adipose stem cells and have an unlimited lifetime supply of their own cells.

When I started my cord blood stem cell storage company, it was still very new in the market and the pushback was actually from the doctors in the hospital who didn't want to be bothered with having to collect the cord blood.

Even though they usually aren't the ones doing it – it's almost always a nurse or medical assistant doing the actual collection – they still didn't like that it was a "new thing" to have to deal with.

I'll never forget the comment from the doctor who delivered our first child, regarding our collection of cord blood. "If we have time, we'll try to get to your science experiment." He referred to it as a frivolous science experiment and was annoyed that he had to be bothered with it. He was an older doctor and likely was not ready for this new world of advanced stem cell therapy.

A few years later I spoke to the partner in that same obstetrics office, and he said they had seen multiple children whose lives had been saved by cord blood banking and he was now an advocate for cord blood storage.

His partner had mocked it only a few years before that, then suddenly it hit them that it's not just a science experiment, but an advanced lifesaving medical protocol. Suddenly, the world they worked in was new and different, and people who previously would not have been alive were now alive because of it. It happened that fast.

I continued that lab venture into medical school but had to hand it off to a colleague due to time constraints: med school is pretty busy. I was halfway through medical school when I was invited to co-venture and open a biotech lab focusing on stem cell processing and stem cell product manufacture for medical use by physicians in the orthopedic and pain management space.

I took a leave of absence from medical school to be the chief science and medical officer for this biotech venture and opened this new biotech lab in Arizona, one of the hubs of biotech in the nation at that time.

I was already through the academics of medical school, and I realized two things pretty quickly. Firstly, what I was being taught was so far behind what I had already studied in biotech that if I wanted to be at the forefront of medical innovation, I would not get there by traditional medical school processes for at least a decade.

Secondly, I could do so much more good in the medical world through my experience in biotechnology and business than I would finishing medical school and going into residency for several more years.

I saw the writing on the wall pretty quickly and chose the path of biotech and innovation. I'll forever be grateful for the medical knowledge I gained from my academic years in medical school; this education has greatly helped me in the process.

I'll always advocate for education, but there's a point where you know what you know, you know what other people don't know, you know what you can do and what other people can't do or aren't doing, and you start seeing the opportunities where you can make a larger impact.

It took several months of contemplation to not go back and finish med school, but my path was already being structured for me through successful efforts in this new biotech venture I'd left med school for. I never looked back, and I have directly seen my positive impact at the national level in the field of regenerative medicine.

I built a tissue processing lab in Arizona and developed multiple product lines and lectured on stem cells and clinical applications at multiple medical conferences before my med school colleagues were finished with school.

As of the time of writing, I have started multiple biotech companies, multiple medical companies, built/owned/operated multiple clinical labs, developed dozens of products and services in the medical field, and written hundreds of pages of scientifically backed content for these operations and for product use in the medical field.

I have also written numerous treatment protocols for the application of regenerative medicine products in medical practice, and I've personally taught and coached hundreds of physicians and medical providers on the use and application of biologic products and many other aspects of the field of regenerative medicine, resulting in the direct application of therapy to tens of thousands of patients.

I would say that one of my greater achievements in this space has been the education, coaching, and awareness I've brought to hundreds of physicians around the nation. This has probably done more to advance regenerative medicine than anything else I could have done during those years after I left medical school.

I'm excited to bring this guidebook to you for your personal education on your options for the various regenerative medicine treatments available in the United States and in the international medical field.

Let's dive in!

Chapter 1: Stem Cells

Stem Cells 101

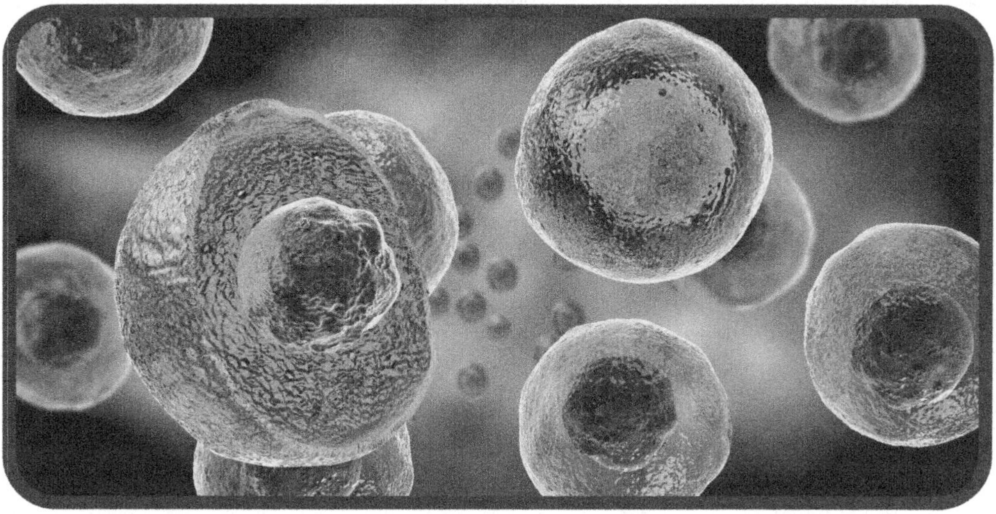

A stem cell is the foundation unit of cellular growth and development. It's basically a blank slate cell that can grow in any direction it needs for cellular development of the whole body.

The remarkable behavior of a stem cell is that when it divides into two cells, one cell will divert off into the type of cell it needs to become, and the remaining cell stays a stem cell and can split again and again to produce more and more cells as needed.

This process of a stem cell splitting into a new specialized type of cell is called differentiation - the process of becoming different. It's a nice scientific word for a stem cell changing into a different cell type, and you'll hear it a lot because it's the fundamental aspect of what makes stem cells so amazing; the secret sauce of why stem cells are so useful.

Stem cells replicate and differentiate over and over and over. This is where it really gets interesting. How long can this go on? How long can stem cells keep dividing and creating a new dedicated cell line while the original one stays a stem cell?

Turns out, basically your whole life, though it slows down and there are DNA mechanisms for how long it can do this, called telomeres and most people have started hearing about these in recent years.

Telomeres are the ends of a DNA strand and are the most commonly discussed aspect of cellular replication because telomere length can determine how many times a cell can replicate. This makes it an attractive subject to study, because being able to control this process may make it possible to control cellular replication capabilities over long periods of time.

Telomeres don't code for things, like physical features and such, but they make it possible for the rest of the DNA to work. This replication declining mechanism has been identified as, and believed to be, a source and ultimate cause of aging and age-related illnesses.

Simply put, telomeres measure our life span and capacity to age and die. As just mentioned, a telomere is the extra end string of DNA left over after a cell has replicated its DNA. The easiest way to describe a telomere is this: you tie a shoestring, but you don't tie the knot at the very end, you tie it down where the strings meet the braid.

You then have nice long strings left over. You need that long string in order to tie another knot, because you can't tie a good knot using a short string. Also, you still need a nice tight knot with no dangling strands, so you cut off the extra length of string hanging off that knot. That's how telomeres get shorter with each replication cycle, they are clipped off to keep the DNA coil nice and tight with no "loose ends."

Over time, each replication shaves a little DNA off the end of that string, so eventually there's no telomere string left to tie knots with, but you still must tie those knots with every replication cycle, so you start tying knots with actual DNA that codes for important things. Afterall, there's plenty of string left, it's just string that is actual DNA sequences the code for things. So you don't want to start chopping those pieces off!

That DNA is now being chopped off the ends as well, just like telomeres were before, and you start losing valuable DNA. This is the beginning of the end of that DNA strand. After a while, that shoe is barely hanging on and will most likely fall off with a little too much activity.

This simplified description helps explain how telomeres are associated with stem cell activity. The question of how long a stem cell can replicate is a bit more complex, but it's really easy to understand that there is a limit. Now you know two terms: differentiation and telomeres. You're on your way to being a stem cell expert!

The entire story of stem cells is a little more than I want to get into in this book, but what I do want to discuss is the category of stem cells that is currently applicable to medical use. These two basic concepts of differentiation and telomeres really summarize why we need stem cells in medicine.

After a while, you just aren't going to make enough cells fast enough to replace the aging/dying/damaged cells in your body, and that is why everyone should be extremely excited about the new field of stem cell medicine. This is also why I believe that routine infusions of our own cultured expanded stem cells could be the key to system-wide health and longevity. More on this later!

You obviously want to learn about the tremendous advantages stem cell therapies have for average medical conditions. After all, this is a guidebook to stem cell therapy for specific medical conditions associated with respiratory health that you're interested in learning about, so it makes sense that I get to brass tacks on this.

Stem Cell Types

Hematopoietic stem cells: (he-mat-o-poi-et-ic) Hematopoietic stem cells differentiate into blood-based cells. Heme is the medical scientific word for iron, and the medical word for anything to do with blood, because iron makes your blood red and transports oxygen.

For example, hematology is the study of blood, so that should help you remember that hematopoietic stem cells make your blood cells. Most stem cell therapies you'll hear about in the coming years are NOT hematopoietic based therapies, and that's why I wanted to mention them first and then put them aside while I get to the more popular and more diverse category of mesenchymal stem cells.

Mesenchymal stem cells: (mess-en-ky-mal) Mesenchymal stem cells differentiate into many other cell types. One of these types is musculoskeletal tissue, also known medically as MSK.

MSK tissue contains cells such as cartilage, bone, muscle, tendons, and connective tissues, which are of particular interest in regenerative medicine because there are so many conditions in this category that can be treated.

You need to remember the initialism MSK because this is what is used most of the time to describe this category. This means mesenchymal stem cells are the type that can regenerate tissues for all the various injuries we endure through the daily activities of life.

Everything from spinal stenosis and osteoarthritis to serious spinal injuries would look to mesenchymal stem cells as a possible treatment.

In order to explain the treatment possibilities with mesenchymal stem cells, there are two more terms I want to teach you here: autologous and allogeneic. Autologous means it comes from you; allogeneic means it comes from someone else and is given to you. These two terms define the entire state of stem cell therapy in the US and internationally.

See, you are really becoming a stem cell expert because most people have no idea those two terms exist or what they mean, much less that those two terms are how the world of stem cell therapy is divided up.

What is and what is not an actual stem cell treatment?

Buckle in and I'll run through a snap account of the regenerative medicine product portfolio in the market today. I'll follow up after this on where you're likely to see and hear about these different products and therapies, what to look for, and what to avoid.

Stem Cell Treatments and Products

The first thing you have to know is that the term "stem cells" accidentally became a common vernacular term for any regenerative product because it was the preferred term to use. This is because it was such a high-end medical term and because there were so many different products, it was hard to explain the differences, so everyone just called everything stem cells.

This caused a lot of confusion and, ultimately, got the attention of the FDA and the FTC; I'll explain those details later.

Bone marrow stem cells for MSK use: (autologous) Bone marrow stem cells are collected from your own bone marrow, processed, refined and concentrated, and reinjected into the target treatment areas. The combination of cells in this bone marrow collection are excellent at regenerating damaged tissues. This is considered the traditional standard stem cell treatment in the US, and has been the standard for stem cells treating musculoskeletal conditions for the last couple of decades.

The downsides are that it requires a very uncomfortable procedure to collect bone marrow aspirate stem cells (BMAC), and the cells are technically as old as you are, so that whole section on telomeres now starts to make sense; your own stem cells are not any younger than you are.

Note on growing stem cells

There's a caveat to the cells being "as old as you are" and a misconception that because they are as old as you that they aren't going to provide as much benefit as cells from a birth tissue stem cell product. There are several reasons why this isn't all the way true, and it's been blown out of proportion by all the companies that make birth tissue biologic products.

They'd love for all of you to believe that the only cells worth having are age 0 stem cells from birth tissues like placenta tissue, amniotic membrane, cord tissues, and Wharton's Jelly and such. The reality is that there are more aspects to consider than just the age of the cells.

One of the more interesting bodies of knowledge coming out of the stem cell research world is that when you culture and expand, grow and replicate stem cells in the lab, they turn into very active cells. There are multiple articles out there showing that adult stem cells that are triggered to culture expand and replicate at the same metabolic rates as brand new age 0 cells.

It's a very interesting phenomenon that means that adult stem cell replication is a very viable option. This means that adults can have their cells cultured into nearly unlimited doses of viable stem cells that can be used the rest of their lives!

Adipose stem cells: Adipose stem cells are stem cells collected from your fat tissue through a liposuction procedure. These are becoming more popular for several reasons, and I'll explain how this might be the best option for the immediate future of stem cell therapy in the US.

To recap how this process works, first a small lipoaspirate procedure is performed, effectively a small liposuction procedure. It's only a 40-60ml collection of lipoaspirate, so it's a very small amount compared to what a plastic surgeon might normally collect in one of their procedures.

The procedure itself is very quick, maybe 10min, and relatively painless and only requires local anesthesia on the tissue area. It's quick, painless, and affordable. The result is a collection of ideal adipose tissue that can now produce all the stem cells you'll need for the rest of your life!

The lipoaspirate is then sent to the lab, the cells are isolated and characterized, meaning we identify the stem cells specifically, and then those specific stem cells are cultured and expanded, meaning they are grown and replicated into numerous vials of millions and millions of cells.

Literally, you can produce more stem cells than you'll ever need in a lifetime of regular treatment, so this is clearly the most effective and efficient way to engage in long-term stem cell treatment plans.

I'm a very strong advocate for this procedure because I believe it will be the most effective and accessible stem cell treatment modality in the coming years, especially with the current legal climate on stem cells. My company Longevity Stem Cells is poised to be the nation's premier stem cell collection and storage bank in the nation and I'm excited to promote it. You can learn about what we are about in this link: www.longevitystemcells.com.

For years, adipose stem cells were a battleground for regenerative medicine advocates because the FDA claimed that the resulting stem cells produced from a collection procedure effectively constituted a product that entered the market and was then offered to the patient as a treatment.

So the FDA wanted to intervene and control that process. Treating the stem cells collected from an individual's adipose tissue, and reinjected back into the patient, as a biologic drug that requires trials and pharmaceutical grade regulation would have effectively made this an impossible hurdle in the stem cell world.

Luckily, about two years ago, a federal court case in California ruled that the relationship between a doctor and a patient in which an adipose collection and stem cell treatment was performed was a medical procedure in the office agreed to by both physician and patient and did not fall under the purview of the FDA and did not constitute a product that entered the market.

This meant that the FDA no longer had a legal standing to intervene in the adipose stem cell treatment process. This was a huge win for the stem cell industry, the true and legitimate stem cell industry.

Remember, even a product that works extremely well can fail if the people using it make unsubstantiated claims, are abusive in their marketing tactics, or are abusive in pricing the treatment. Something to consider is that this option requires a small liposuction to collect the fat and harvest the cells, so it's still a little invasive, but not nearly as invasive as bone marrow collections.

Cultured expanded stem cells – Autologous and Allogeneic: This is my favorite category of stem cell treatment because it's THE future of stem cell therapy worldwide.

Cultured and expanded stem cells are grown in specialized cell culture labs and can be grown using autologous or allogeneic stem cells. So you can use your bone marrow stem cells and grow them out to get a proper high dose for treatment, or you can use ethical and compliant perinatal tissue stem cells. You can isolate and grow a tremendous quantity of specific mesenchymal stem cells and have enough for multiple treatments all at the same time.

I'll take a moment to say that I used to promote the idea that these expanded cell therapies were only available outside of the US. For cultured birth tissue stem cells this is still the case, but you can have your own adipose stem cells harvested, cultured, and expanded for your own personal use here in the US. This opens the door to a wide range of treatment options here in the US that don't require international travel.

Most of what people are looking for with international travel and treatment is all available here in the US, they just aren't aware of it or their doctors are not aware of how to access it. I also believe a lot of doctors and medical companies have invested heavily in international treatment centers that they are obligated to refer to, so it would be hard to get them to change their patterns. The best option may be to find a doctor who'll do these treatments here rather than coerce or pressure you into traveling to a foreign nation to get a shady unknown stem cell treatment just because they own a small fraction of that treatment center!

Same day treatment versus culture expanded cells? Ultimate problem with bone marrow or adipose cells offered as same day treatment is that you can only get so much material, only so many stem cells and beneficial material available in a single collection, so you can only create enough high dose stem cell content for limited use. Cell expansion is the future of stem cell treatment because you can grow as much as you need or want.

For a person considering these options, consider this – you'll likely need more than one treatment for the same thing. There is almost never a one-and-done scenario with regen med. You'll need to do another treatment eventually, and that will mean another harvesting procedure that you don't want to go through.

With advanced cell culturing techniques, we can grow as many vials of cells as you'll ever need in your life. It's certainly worth it to engage in one adipose collection event so you can obtain stem cells for the rest of your life!

The culture expansion capabilities of a single collection ensure that you could supply yourself with hundreds of doses of your own cells for the rest of your life, which will likely be longer now that you're engaging in regular stem cell therapies for many of your issues.

Back to the beauty of how stem cells work in the culture setting. One of the benefits of stem cells that will be very useful down the road is to differentiate those cells into specific tissue type cells. Think of growing a batch of cardiac stem cells specifically for heart repair, or a batch of cartilage tissue stem cells for joint injuries! Also, think: lab grown organs and tissues.

This is THE advantage in stem cell medicine and therapy and the future of cellular medicine as it becomes more formalized and standardized for predictable outcomes, and this will be possible through culture expansion work to grow these cells into what we need them to be.

Culture and expansion from a single collection/harvesting event is much more efficient than having to engage in an autologous collection event like bone marrow or adipose collection procedures every time you want to get a treatment. The reason we see so much bone marrow and adipose activity in the US is because doctors are used to offering same day treatment after harvesting and rarely work with patients to culture/expand and bank their cells for later use.

Culturing and expanding birth tissue cells, however, is still an off limits category and it would still require international travel to get treatment with this category. This is mostly for good reasons though, as it's very complicated to get it right and it needs to be refined and standardized for wide-scale application.

This is where the stem cell research field comes in line with large pharmaceutical companies. They are working on more formal cellular therapies that qualify as biologic drugs, so as they continue their research we'll see more advances.

Standardizing cellular therapy is not like other manufactured medications or treatments where chemistry can replicate the same molecule perfectly. Cell culture is like trying to encourage the cells to replicate the way you want, but you can't always count on it to be a perfect replication process.

This is why it's hard to regulate cultured cell therapies, but the industry is getting much better at these processes, AND the doctors I've talked to are much more willing by far to offer treatment using the patient's own stem cells versus any other source.

I've also asked the question to many doctors if they'd be willing to offer treatment to patients who have had their own adipose stem cells cultured and expanded. They have all said yes to this as well because they believe that if it's the patient's own cells it's an acceptable treatment.

I intend to be a part of the cellular therapy standardization process in the US because it's definitely the future of medicine, but I don't want it to be in a field that is bombarded with bad actors trying to game the market.

As of this writing, I am working with my team on some of these standardized cultured expanded stem cell therapies with plans and hopes to conduct trials and help get these treatments through the approval process in the US.

At any time while reading this book, you can reach out to me and I'll direct you to some of the best options for this around the world. will@willbozeman.com and I'll connect you to the right people and companies that can help get you started!

Obviously, the MSK category is already a highly popular category, but now we are seeing movement into treatments for things like COPD (chronic obstructive pulmonary disease), heart tissue repair, neural tissue repair, eye and ocular healing and repair, advanced esthetics and hair regeneration, and, of course, one of my favorites, longevity and anti-aging therapies through full-body inflammation reduction via IV stem cell therapy.

There are a lot of other really exciting things, but I don't want to suggest that these conditions are being cured with these stem cell treatments yet. Some treatment types are helping these people and, in many cases, it's about the only available option that will work, even if it's a modest result.

I personally knew a retired medical doctor who sought stem cell IV treatment for his chronic condition. I don't want to say what it was because I don't want to suggest that what he did will work for anyone else, nor that cultured expanded cell therapy will treat or cure this particular condition or act as a treatment option just yet, but he had very impressive results and I almost didn't believe it.

Unfortunately, this treatment only curbed the symptoms, which is still amazing for what it was able to do for him, and he'd have to get another treatment to maintain the effects. This is why I'm such a proponent of banking your own supply of stem cells for the rest of your life! His condition came back eventually, but the severity of his symptoms was significantly reduced and mostly resolved for nearly a year after that treatment. He didn't go get another treatment because he would have to travel internationally and pay tens of thousands of dollars again for treatment.

I can think of many people and many conditions where if there was a routine annual stem cell treatment that only reduced the severity of the symptoms, it would still be a tremendous success and would become the new standard of care for that condition. Everyone should have their own banked supply!

His results were something I didn't believe would happen at all. I knew the guy decently well; he was a retired family practice doctor. So our conversations on his treatment process were very interesting. He made me believe that what they are saying they're able to do in the international stem cell treatment market is actually possible using cultured expanded stem cell therapies.

Now I have seen this exact treatment occur here in the US under the right circumstances, so I know it's possible to manage these conditions with your own cells.

I know it's exciting, but it's still a very new field, so I'm not suggesting or claiming that any condition I mention or discuss is curable or can be cured with these treatments … yet. I simply believe it is the right track to a better future of medical treatment.

Birth tissue stem cell products: Immediately, I want to point out that the birth tissue stem cell products I'm talking about here come from perfectly ethical and legally donated tissues that come from normal, healthy Cesarean section deliveries by donors who are fully informed about the procedure and go through rigorous and regulated vetting, screening, and testing.

I know a lot about this process as I've launched multiple companies and labs that made these birth-tissue-based regenerative products. The best way to think of how this is compliant and moral and ethical is to understand that during a regular C-section delivery, the mother and the baby are safe and healthy and they both move on with their lives as normal, but what about all the leftover birth tissues involved in the process?

Those tissues are normally disposed of as medical waste, but they are perfectly healthy tissues that can be repurposed into something useful. This is exactly what the perinatal birth tissue category has accomplished, using healthy, safe tissues that are safely, ethically, and morally collected and processed into useful medical products. It's a wonderful way to make something useful out of something that would otherwise be useless.

All the collection programs I worked with in my career were heavily regulated by the FDA and a very detailed paper trail was in place for each tissue collection we received. I've explained the appropriateness of this category of tissue collection to hundreds of doctors and patients.

Everyone is skeptical after hearing about some of the bad actors in the industry mentioned in news articles. I'd be skeptical, too, if I hadn't actually been in the middle of this process for so long. I've seen so much good come from this treatment category, and, of course, where there's good there's going to be a few bad actors exploiting that good.

There is a range of products created from perinatal birth tissues. Two of the primary reasons birth tissues are so useful are: first, the cells are brand new, so they are young and active and have a full life cycle of replication potential, if you recall the topic of telomeres and stem cell replication lifespan.

The second reason is that the cells in the tissues have little to no detectable immunomarkers on the cells. This means that you don't have to type match a donor to a recipient like you do with blood and organs. I've explained this concept to several hundred doctors over my biotech career because, to the average trained physician, our cells have markers that identify ourselves versus foreign cells.

The short answer to why these tissues have little to no detectable immunomarkers is that the mother and the developing baby are two unique entities with their own identifying immunity markers. So if they could sense each other's presence, they'd fight each other with their own immune responses.

Birth tissues like the placenta, umbilical cord, and amniotic membrane are created specifically to overcome this problem by being immune marker neutral tissues. The amniotic fluid, membrane, umbilical cord, and placenta are designed to shield the two entities from each other, thus making the tissues ideal for use as stem cell sources because the cells won't have immune markers to trigger responses.

Here's a list of the different birth tissues that are popular for stem cell collection:

Industry note:

At the time of writing, all birth tissue injectable biologics are being reclassified under FDA regulations, so you may not see many of these in the market anymore until regulators iron out how they will be allowed moving forward.

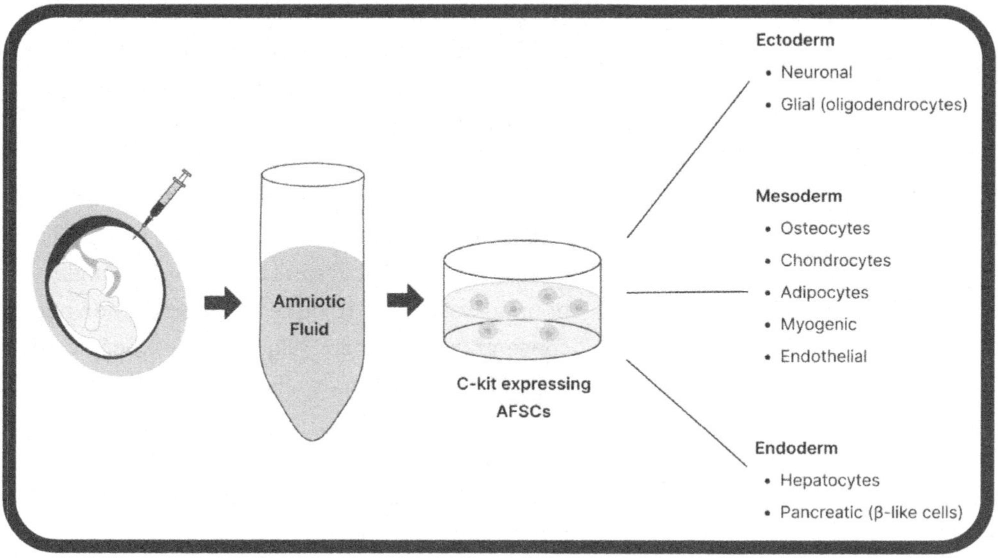

Amniotic fluid stem cell isolation and differentiation.

Data from: https://www.researchgate.net/figure/Amniotic-fluid-stem-cell-AFSC-isolation-and-differentiation-Cells-are-collected-via_fig1_342967332

Amniotic fluid stem cells: This is the actual fluid that the fetus floated in and lived in during development. Naysayers love to claim this is just baby urine, but I've only ever heard this argument when a doctor is trying to sell you what they're offering, that isn't amniotic fluid.

Also, with all the studies on amniotic fluid in recent years, they've been proven wildly incorrect over the last decade for trying to suggest that amniotic fluid is mere baby urine. Again, they're only saying that if they're trying to sell you something else.

Whether intentionally selling something else or unintentionally, due to lack of education on the details, it's not the same world we lived in 20 years ago when it comes to understanding biologics.

Though it's true that babies do "urinate" a mild diluted version of urine in amniotic fluid, they also continuously drink amniotic fluid as well because it is completely safe for the fetus to consume, and this fluid is filled with high levels of a wide range of growth factors and nutrients. It's nature's perfect regenerative fluid.

Remember that the baby's actual harmful waste is removed through the mother via the umbilical cord, not via the baby, so all the harmful elements of urine waste have to be removed so they do not concentrate in the baby's liquid waste where it would build up to dangerous levels in amniotic fluid.

So, if you hear "baby urine," then you know you're being sold, or the doctor isn't very solid on their regen med background.

However, I like to look at it as an opportunity to learn and grow. After all, I taught hundreds of doctors a wide range of regen med topics over the years that helped them apply therapies to patients. They have to start somewhere, and most of the time the doctors I taught were starting from scratch. I applaud them for leaping into the future!

Will's Industry Insight #1:
Ultimately, after 30,000+ cases using products created in my labs throughout my biotech career, the general consensus from the doctors and practices I've worked with is that fresh frozen amniotic fluid works better and produces better and longer outcomes.

Amniotic fluid comes in two main forms: fresh frozen and room temperature sterilized. I've worked with many versions of both and seen amazing outcomes with both for many years.

Will's Industry Insight #2:
Genuine amniotic fluid is not considered a stem cell product, yet it has been routinely called stem cells as a commonly used vernacular term by doctors and pretty much everyone else in the industry. Now you can see how easy it is to confuse the different names of treatments and confuse patients on what they're getting.

There may be a few viable stem cells in fresh amniotic fluid by the time it's injected into a patient, but nowhere near enough to justify calling it a stem cell injection, not to mention that many amniotic fluid products intentionally screen out the cell content.

Also, when a doctor or medical office says their frozen ready to go product has "millions of stem cells," they're talking about general cell content, NOT stem cell counts.

What percentage of cells in these tissues are actual stem cells? It varies, but in amniotic fluid, for example, about 2-3% of the cell content is actual stem cells; the rest are all sorts of other tissue cells. In the US, we are not allowed to refine and concentrate stem cells out of birth tissues into a concentrated injection, so if the doctor is taking a vial out of the freezer, you're not getting a vial full of stem cells, you're getting a vial full of a homogenous tissue composed of mostly non-stem cells and tissue particulates, an injection with very few stem cells that most likely will not be viable living healthy cells by the time they are injected.

Will's Industry Insight #3:
"Is my doctor selling me a certain number of cells?" If you're in the US then the short answer is no, not really, at least not really stem cells. Again, being a biotech founder, product developer, and manufacturer, and working closely with hundreds of doctors gives you a lot of insight into how easy it is to misunderstand what the product is and how to describe it to a patient.

So, you can see how this is misleading if a medical office is advertising stem cell treatments and claims to have high quantities of stem cells in the injection. That's outright misleading and that's what has gotten the attention of the FDA and gotten the Federal Trade Commission, FTC, involved in regulating what doctors say to patients and what biotech labs and sales reps say to doctors.

Despite the lack of genuine stem cell quantities in ready-to-go products in the US market, here's the real kicker you won't hear from your doctor or medical office: pure acellular amniotic fluid works as well as or better than cellular-based injections … without any cell content!

You won't hear that from the office trying to sell you a treatment based on stem cell counts or stem cell viability content, but I've seen and heard this many times in offices that do a lot of treatment volume. This is what actually led me to create an acellular product line in the first place – to make a pure amniotic fluid product with no cell content. It worked tremendously well and outperformed a wide range of other products that claimed to have cell content.

As I mentioned before, if it's in the US and they're advertising an allogeneic stem cell product, aka a frozen, ready-to-go injection taken out of the freezer, with a specified cell count, they are not being honest with you about what you're buying, or the doctors themselves are not aware of what they are selling.

Either way, you're not getting what you think you're getting. Aside from that, the assumption for years was that the relatively few viable stem cells in the product were what produced the amazing outcomes everyone was seeing.

Despite the debate over cell content, most doctors I've worked with claim they see as good or better outcomes with pure fluid with no cell content. So, you can see that cells or no cells, it works. So it really does matter what the doctor is selling you and that you're aware of what you're paying for.

But for your own peace of mind, that product you did get injected with will probably work well and these nuances won't really matter. It just helps shape the background of the industry we are in to understand all these details.

t

Unfortunately, it's too easy to just call everything stem cells, but I believe once you attach a price to that stem cell quantity claim you're making, you have to be able to verify that claim, and doctors can't do that in the office, nor can the labs do that once it's in the doctor's office and out of the lab setting. Call it what it is and let the results speak for themselves because the results are still great, they just need to get the messaging right.

Will's Industry Insight #4:
They all work about the same anyway! Most birth tissue products have roughly the same outcomes, despite what tissue they're derived from, or the cell counts, or anything else. I've talked to many doctors about this, and they all agree that the outcome differences between one type and another are nominal, meaning the differences are nominal, but the outcomes are good across the board.

So … why the range of products? The ability to make a different product and stand out in the biotech market is a possibility for any biotech company, so it's attractive to create a unique product rather than just copy another. This was a very common practice for years and created the "Wild West" of new biologic regenerative medicine products.

Will's Industry Insight #5:
Everything your doctor knows about stem cells, they've learned from a sales rep, or at least this was the norm for years and years. It's an unfortunate truth that the vast majority of what you're hearing in the doctor's office was taught by a sales rep for whatever product company is selling the product, and it did not come from medical education or personal research by the doctor.

I've been asked/recruited/petitioned vigorously by multiple labs and startups to help them create unique birth tissue products to take to market. They all want something they can call their own, something unique, something different, ultimately so they can corner the market on that one type of product that is unique to them.

It's not all bad for companies to want something special. It really is the driver of innovation and positive change in this industry. Because of this drive to innovate novel products, we've landed on some amazing products in the market and the possibility that there will be FDA-approved products in the coming years. It's all spurred by competition and the drive to make something new.

Stem cells are such a new field, doctors don't get educated on it in medical school. I know because I asked about it specifically and my med school professors told me it wasn't a viable subject to teach yet because it was so new.

While they were saying those words in class, I was actively developing the product manufacturing process for my first biotech product venture to isolate cell-rich tissues and make injectable products. We were seeing tremendous results with this product all while my professors wouldn't even acknowledge these as viable treatment options.

So where do the doctors learn about it while in practice? Pretty much from the sales reps making rounds in their offices. Now, I won't go into how risky this is, but I know exactly how these companies craft their products and messages to appear better, unique, different, and something extra special, and, in some cases, something that they actually aren't, as I've stated above.

That said, I can tell in about five seconds if a doctor is reciting sales material education to me or if they know what they are talking about. I had my own set of questions I'd ask that would "prove out" the doctor as reciting sales rep info as their own knowledge.

So I can say from experience that most of the doctors I've talked to, who endeavored to be in the regenerative medicine space, learned everything they know about it from sales reps. Don't even get me started on the sales reps and product distributors in the market.

Most of the reps I've talked to couldn't speak to stem cells or regen med beyond what is printed on the brochure. Some of them are earnest and trying to do good and earn a living, others not so much.

I used to indulge these reps when they wanted to sell me on their company's products or try to recruit me to their company, and I've been the secret shopper for doctors trying to learn the details of a product and been on those phone calls or even in the office to hear the pitch and ask the "hard questions" that the rep should know if they know anything at all.

Some of the doctors I've helped have connected with me for years to help them evaluate a new company or product, needing someone to make sense of the confusion in the market for them.

Additionally, the risky part is that these are usually not professional sales reps like salaried employees who speak for the company, but commission-only sales reps who were never actually medically trained, have never operated professionally in the medical space, or, in some cases, never went to college, and here they are "teaching" doctors about stem cell treatments because they have a brochure.

That's why I push for doctors to do their own research and read their own white papers on the subject.

Will's Industry Insight #6:
"My chiropractor said 'stem cells' were reimbursed by Medicare." How many times have I heard this from patients? I stopped keeping count. Hundreds of doctors and chiropractors around the nation billed insurance and Medicare for "stem cell" products that were never reimbursable in the first place.

I've been on dozens of calls to explain why they couldn't do this and what the risk was going to be, and they preferred to believe the commissioned sales rep because what the reps were saying was more exciting ... and profitable. So, no, currently you can't get your stem cells reimbursed by Medicare, and the doctors and chiropractic offices who are telling patients this are incorrect.

I could go into the specific details of why this wasn't allowed, but the short answer is that it's pretty clear in the reimbursement system that there is no reimbursement for unapproved biologics, and if you get reimbursement on it, those payers like Medicare and commercial insurers can come and take that money back from the medical office later, after they figure out that the product and treatment weren't covered.

This is not necessarily a problem for patients to deal with, but it can destroy a medical office if they get all that reimbursement clawed back later, which I've seen many times. So it's just a matter of time. I've literally had dozens of calls with offices and billing companies about the risk of them trying to bill for these products.

I actually pleaded with one doctor who was a friend of mine not to do this. He acted like he'd found this secret success in being able to bill insurances for these treatments. He didn't listen to me.

He got clawed back by multiple insurances all at the same time and he had to shut down his office. It was sad, but I tried my best. Fortunately, one of my other friends took my advice and avoided it. Then he called me a few months later to thank me for keeping him out of all that mess.

Will's Industry Insight #7:
"What's the deal with chiropractors selling stem cells?" Yep, I know it doesn't make sense at all, but I can explain. I'll add a disclaimer to this by saying that many chiropractors don't apply to the following category of activity and that I have good friends who are chiropractors who also bemoan the reputation some chiropractors create in the market on this topic.

Chiropractors are not medical physicians or medical providers, so they need to hire a medical provider to offer medical treatment in their offices.

Years ago, chiropractors discovered that if they hired a genuine medical provider, such as a nurse practitioner (NP), physician assistant (PA), or an actual medical doctor (MD/DO), even just part-time for one day a week, they could effectively operate like a de facto medical office and offer genuine medical treatments instead of only chiropractic adjustments and related work.

In most states, medications, medical therapies, medical procedures like simple injections, and other medical treatments are outside the scope of a chiropractor's license. So, with a part-time medical provider on staff, a chiropractor can now offer all sorts of medical treatments for which they normally are prohibited from engaging in.

So, how did chiropractors get so heavy in the stem cell market when they aren't even allowed to prescribe that treatment or perform the injections?

The short answer is that it was a new, high-end, cash pay medical procedure that actually worked well to relieve pain and, most importantly, it could be administered by a part-time medical provider who came into the office once a week to perform all the procedures that the chiropractor sold to their patients during the week.

With an NP who comes once or twice a week, you can offer all these treatments and schedule them all on the day the NP is on site and operate like a medical office in the eyes of the patient, and in many cases these offices go the extra mile and remove "chiropractic" from the office name to enhance the medical aspect of the office.

A chiropractic office that employs a medical provider is usually called an "integrated chiropractic office," or simply an "integrated office" for short. This model has been very common for the last couple of decades.

In fact, there are whole consulting companies dedicated specifically to coaching chiropractors to appear like medical offices in the market, using this term "integrated medical office," where the intent is to rename your practice to something that doesn't include the term "chiropractor" in the title.

I've seen dozens of chiropractic offices change their names under these consultant groups' instructions. I've asked several of them why they changed the name and removed any reference to chiropractic services and the answers are that they want patients to see them as genuine medical offices with medical treatments, not just chiropractic services, even though the majority of the time the office is open there may not be a medical provider on site at all.

There's nothing wrong with a nurse practitioner working in a chiropractic office in this way, except when it becomes confusing to the patient about who is practicing medicine or who is the medical authority in the office.

A chiropractor is not a medical authority over a genuine medical provider like an NP, PA, or MD/DO, so if a patient is confused about this, it creates problems, yet it's that state of confusion that many chiropractors have counted on in order to sell high-dollar stem cell treatments for years.

Many states are starting to look at this model because if the chiropractor pays the salary of the medical provider, then the medical provider may be incentivized to perform medical services under the direction of the chiropractor, which they are not allowed to do because medical therapies are outside the scope of a chiropractor, and chiropractors are not allowed to dictate the course of medical care to a medical provider.

You can see how this is also confusing for medical providers employed by chiropractors. I've been in many of these offices and I've seen some that kept the appropriate line of authority in place, which is great and perfectly legitimate.

I've also seen offices where the chiropractor operated like a medical doctor, wore a white coat with a stethoscope around their neck, presented themselves like a medical physician, and discussed medical treatments with the patient, and of course sold expensive stem cell treatments.

Now take that confusing environment of selling patients high-dollar stem cell treatments that aren't really stem cell treatments and you have a recipe for consumer fraud. This is what ultimately created the problems we saw in the stem cell treatment market several years ago, leading to wide-scale industry restrictions.

About ten years ago, as of this writing, one company in particular coached hundreds of chiropractic offices on selling high-dollar stem cell treatments. They advertised heavily and made a lot of promises.

One of the popular phrases was "one-and-done," indicating that you only need one injection and the stem cells would heal your tissues and that's all you would ever need. It doesn't work that way with these products and treatments. As I've already described, you'll likely need multiple rounds of the same treatment over time to maintain the positive effects. The underlying condition the patient has is still there. These injections help in many ways but don't cure anything.

This was a huge problem that ultimately led the FDA and the FTC to crack down on unscrupulous offices making all sorts of claims and charging obscene amounts of money to "cure" medical problems using products that aren't actually stem cells.

I'm all about innovation and creativity, and if all this somehow actually helped advance stem cell medicine, I wouldn't complain. But it didn't advance the field, it damaged the reputation of the field and even drove Google and Facebook to ban ads for stem cell therapies under pressure from government regulators ... yes, even for genuine stem cell therapies in legitimate offices, so it hurt everyone and set the whole industry back.

OK, I know I'm probably going a little too deep on this topic, but it's very important to understand this in terms of the condition of the stem cell market in the US because there's a reason you can only get certain types of stem cell therapy here in the US versus what's available around the world. BUT we are moving on in the world of stem cells to bigger and better things.

I just want those reading this to understand that history because I still get this question from people all the time: what's the deal with chiropractors and stem cells? Now you know a little about that.

Will's Industry Insight #8: "
Dose and concentration are everything! A quick note here on dosing, aka cell concentration. Standardization is the key ingredient in the future success of stem cell treatment.

Some companies have been compiling excellent documentation on the standardization of genuine stem cell and platelet-rich plasma (PRP) therapies in the world. And guess what the secret ingredient is for healing success? Dosing!

You have to concentrate the treatment high enough to produce enough stimulation to induce the in-situ cells and tissues to heal. If you don't concentrate the dose, you won't get the outcomes, and there are studies showing just how much concentration is needed to obtain those outcomes.

We are well on our way to standardizing the regenerative medicine world by collecting all this excellent data on concentration and outcomes. For instance, most of the doctors who offer you a PRP injection in their office are only going to be able to concentrate it in a range of three to four times the concentration it naturally occurs in the blood.

What is the concentration needed to start seeing a huge difference in healing effect? Speaking to many providers and reviewing articles, 7x the normal concentration is the critical dose level to initiate efficacy, and 7x to 30x to get certain outcomes for certain tissues. This is all still in development and discovery with advances occurring all the time.

So, MOST doctors offering PRP are not even offering something that works on a significant therapeutic range. So, never make your choice based on price! The office down the street is going to claim to offer PRP cheaper, but they most likely aren't even in the same ballgame. Same for stem cells: you have to concentrate the dose to get the outcome.

That's why I love cultured expanded stem cell therapy, as I mentioned earlier. We can standardize this treatment and grow enough cells to concentrate the dose to create highly effective and successful outcomes. Dose and concentration are everything!

Amniotic membrane stem cells: The amniotic membrane is the actual sac that holds the fetus and fluid. It was one of the first tissues popularized for birth tissue stem cell use. The membrane is ideal because it has one of the lowest levels of immune markers on cell surfaces, nearly undetectable according to some research articles, so the risk of immune responses on recipients would be minimal to negligible.

Amniotic membrane patches: This happens to be an amazing wound care dressing for open wounds. It heals wounds and ulcers that are non-healing or difficult to treat. It's so good and so widely used that it's starting to become a standard of wound care treatment.

Most of these membranes are stripped of their cell content and dehydrated so it's not considered a stem cell product, but I've still heard it described to patients as a stem cell graft or a stem cell patch. It's not. It's just a dried piece of amniotic membrane with a lot of proteins that help tissues grow after being rehydrated on the wound. Still a great product for wound care though!

The amniotic membrane was used for numerous applications as a surgical dressing for burns and as an adjunctive tissue in surgical reconstruction of the oral cavity and bladder, and also for tympanoplasty, arthroplasty, repair of omphaloceles, and prevention of adhesions in pelvic and abdominal surgery.

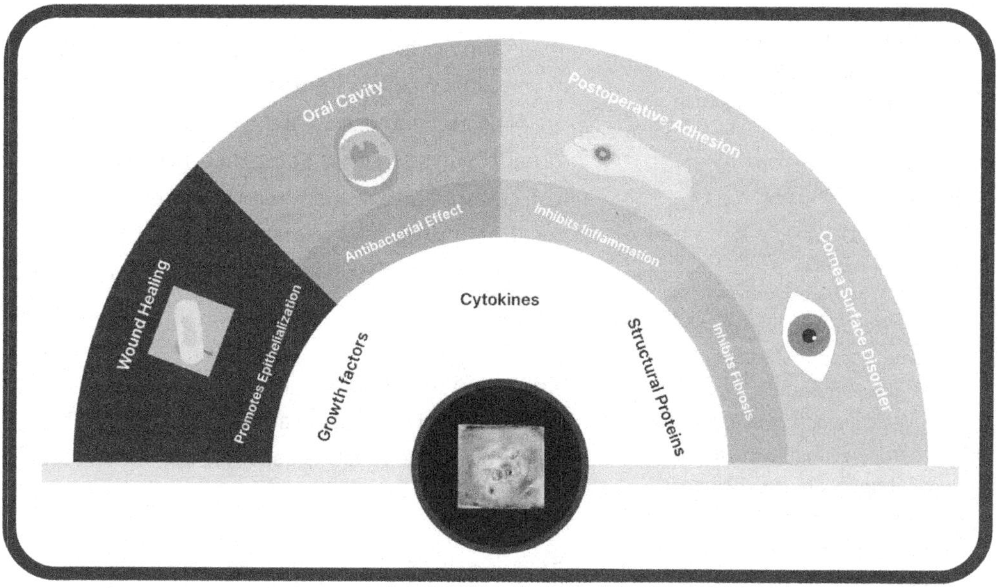

The Amniotic Membrane Is Vital for Medical Applications Like Burn Dressings, Tissue Reconstruction, and Preventing Surgical Adhesions.

Data from: https://www.mdpi.com/2077-0375/11/12/941

Cord blood stem cells: So, if I say blood, you say … hematopoietic. Correct! So, would these cells likely be used in your musculoskeletal treatment? There's a mix of cell types in cord blood, but ultimately cord blood stem cells for general regenerative medicine use and MSK use was heavily scrutinized a few years ago by the FDA and most of those operations were shut down quickly.

Labs were trying to find "the next best thing" to make and sell, but blood products are more complicated because they require blood type matching to be used, or they require more processing work to make them useful, so ultimately you only see cord blood stem cells in high-end medical research therapies like treating various cancers and organ damage.

It's a very exciting category of stem cells, but not the pathway of musculoskeletal treatment that I'm talking about here.

Will's Industry Insight #9: "
Cord tissue stem cells were popularized by a few companies looking to make something different from the more popular amniotic membrane products at the time, eight to 10 years ago.

What I know for certain, because I indirectly caused some of this required innovation, was that various researchers had non-compete contracts that prohibited them from working with amniotic membrane for any new company they worked for, so when those scientists left and worked for another company, or started their own labs, they couldn't work with amniotic membrane and instead worked with cord tissue.

Cord tissue stem cells: This is the umbilical cord itself and all the tissue that makes it up. There's a good bit of cell content in this tissue that can be collected and used. Lately, it's been used as a great tissue source for doing mesenchymal stem cell culture and expansion work in international treatment programs, as the FDA in the US has clamped down on the injectable cord tissue product category.

Collecting the genuine mesenchymal cells out of this tissue for cell replication and expansion is probably going to be the most valuable aspect of this tissue category in the future.

They then had to create the industry perception that cord tissue was "better" or "newer" or "more advanced" than amniotic membrane, when there was no evidence of any superior quality other than that they could actually work with that tissue type under contract. (Just a little insight into why there are so many different product types on the market.)

Yes, I've been involved in conversations with a lot of these labs and companies when they were starting and I've been offered a lot of positions and partnerships and all sorts of things to come over and help these new ventures get off the ground. So I know some of these very intimate industry insights.

Wharton's Jelly stem cells: Wharton's Jelly is the gelatinous cushion that surrounds the vessels in the umbilical cord. It's rich in cell content and is a great tissue category to work with.

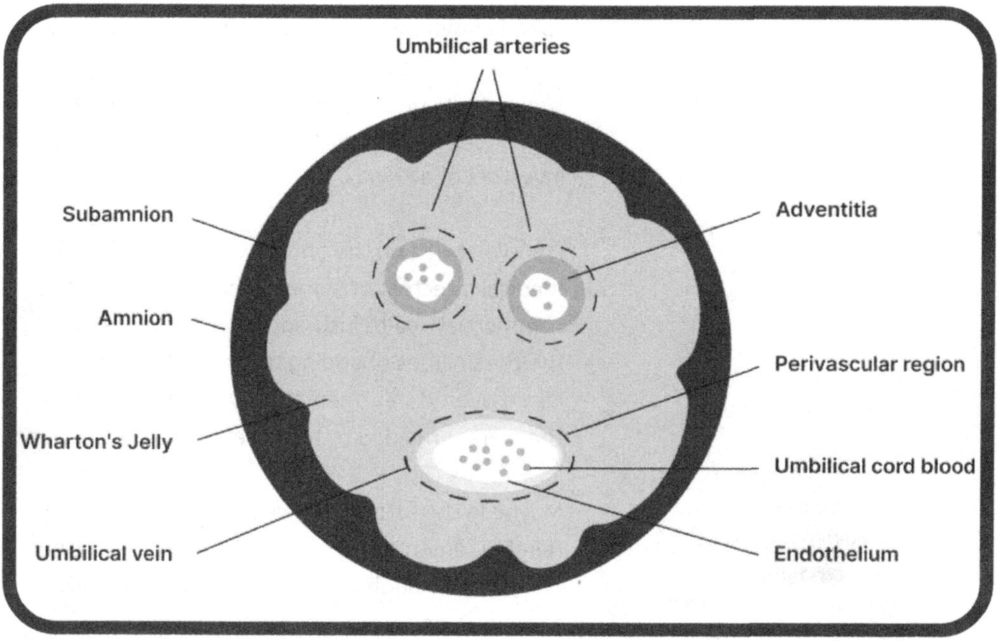

Cross-sectional diagram of a human umbilical cord showing its anatomical compartments, including Wharton's jelly, as a source of stem cells.

Data from: https://www.ncbi.nlm.nih.gov/pmc/articles/PMC3709752/

Often, people use the terms "cord tissue" and "Wharton's Jelly" interchangeably, and although there are differences between them, they are both still great tissues for this industry. Again, we still can't do injections of products like these in the US anymore, but for a while, they were very popular. It's also commonly used in research and for cell culture and expansion.

Placental stem cells: The placenta is another source of cells, but for reasons of complexity I won't go into more detail, but it's still a tissue type you see used in some capacity.

Whew! That's a lot of info for a short run through. I could literally talk about each one of these categories all day. I used to do this all the time: spend endless hours researching and reading all about the cellular biology of all these tissues and spend hours on the phone explaining these details to doctors, labs, other biotech startup groups, and investors of all kinds.

I've even been on the phone with the CEOs and medical directors of some of the top four major commercial health insurance companies discussing the possibilities of adding these product types to their covered treatments. They loved the idea, but the market needed to be more established for them.

Maybe in the future, but we're not there yet on reimbursement for these products. They were very interested though, and I had multiple calls with these groups and spent hours going over the fine details of these different products and the minutiae of differences between them.

I ultimately played the part of an expert witness to their legal departments over the risk of adding these products to their covered services because ultimately it was their legal department that vetoed the use of these products as covered benefits.

They loved hearing about the outcomes and cost efficiency of reducing surgeries and invasive procedures by using these products. I'm sure I'll talk to them again one day when the market is ready for it.

Will's Industry Insight #10: " *Minutiae of differences! Yep, as you can tell from the explanation above, there are a lot of minute details and differences between all these products. To make it even more complex, the FDA had categories to put all these products into and even those categories were nearly impossible for companies to interpret and distinguish.*

Even today I hear of companies trying to make the case that their product is compliant in one category or another when, at the time of writing, the FDA has basically said none of these perinatal tissue products can be sold without now going through a drug trial, except amniotic membrane for wound covering. That's actually still a go and is reimbursable by Medicare and such, but everything else is non-compliant.

Even the companies making these products couldn't explain why their product wasn't the same as another or given the same status.

I had one company's executive team attempt to debate me on how their product was compliant, and I said to them, "I don't need to argue with you, I just need to see your FDA product compliance document – the paper that says your product is compliant under the category you're arguing about."

They couldn't do it, and they were really angry that I knew how to pin them down on this. In most of their sales conversations, they can simply obfuscate the details enough to where the doctor just stops asking questions and believes them.

I don't mince words with these groups anymore because they still damage and discredit the market. I tell them that just because they make a product following the guidelines of that category does not mean it's compliant in that category, and claiming to be compliant and collecting money from sales based on that claim is fraud.

That usually causes them all to pause for a few moments. I'm aiming for a real future in stem cell therapy so I can't suffer the fools who make us all look bad.

Stem cells are a pretty easy term to regulate, so the FDA basically said anyone claiming to offer stem cell treatments or injections is in violation, so they simply track down all the ads and websites claiming stem cells.

Will's Industry Insight #11: " *Stem cells are a dirty word, and it's because of all the charlatans out there! The regulations have now shifted to what you can't say, based on the abuse of all the common terms or words used to describe them.*

Remember that what a doctor or chiropractor's office claims is stem cells that they pull out of the freezer is not stem cells nor is it necessarily what they say it is. It's most likely homogenized tissue injection that may contain a few viable stem cells at best, but it would be misleading to call it a stem cell injection, so regulations had to be enacted.

Doctors and chiropractors would often change to another term to sell the same thing, so each new sales tactic resulted in another restricted word in the market. I've seen the progression of prohibited words keep going and going.

The latest advertisement I saw for a company selling products to doctors' offices called their product "a beneficial injection," using that term because no other word was allowed. So, the advertisement encouraged doctors to call and learn more about what this beneficial injection does for their patients.

"Our beneficial injection is the best beneficial injection on the market." You can see how bad it's gotten when these companies can't use "stem cells" or any other birth tissue name, can't use "regenerative medicine," can't say anything that indicates it's a biologic and are reduced to just calling it a "beneficial injection."

It's pretty comical in some respects, but speaks to how all the bad actors out there have ruined the market. Stem cells are a dirty word now, but my goal is to bring a real and regulated stem cell therapy to the US medical field.

If you are unsure what you've been presented or sold in a doctor's office or chiropractic office please reach out to me and tell me what the product name was and I'll be able to tell you very quickly what the actual material was that was injected or sold to you. Reach out to me at will@willbozeman.com

Chapter 2 - Non-Stem-Cell Products

(Primarily used in the US market)

So, what about non-stem cell products and treatments? There are a lot of them, and I'll run through them quickly. They are not the same thing as any of these above stem cell type therapies, but they do work, and most likely some of these therapies will be the first to market as FDA-approved therapies that get covered by Medicare and commercial insurance companies.

Acellular amniotic fluid – pure fluid: Pure acellular amniotic fluid is amazing as a non-stem cell product. Its outcomes are excellent and it's a very simple product to make and standardize. There are no stem cells to worry about, so you don't have to count cells or worry about viability, which means you don't have to validate or prove cell counts and viability in the lab process.

And remember what I said before: most doctors say their outcomes are roughly as good or even better with pure fluid versus a cellular-based product. Remember all the reasons I mentioned before why a cellular product isn't what you think it is. Pure amniotic fluid is rich in growth factors and nutrients, and other beneficial things.

This chart below shows various research articles describing what cells and tissues have been cultured using amniotic membrane stem cells. Again, very exciting times for medical advancement!

Author, year (Ref)	Regenerated tissue	Treatment
Kajiwara *et al.*, 2017, Kunisaki, 2018 (67, 69)	Fetal	Congenital diaphragmatic hernia, abdominal wall defects, spina bifida, and congenital heart
Cipriani *et al.*, 2007 (68)	Peripheral and central nervous	Neurodegenerative disease such as cerebral ischemia
Di Baldassarre *et al* ., 2018 (70)	Cardiac	Cardiomyoplasty
Chun *et al.*, 2014 (71)	Skeletal muscle	Duchenne muscular dystrophy
Carraro *et al.*, 2008 (72)	Lung	Lung-related disorders such as COVID-19
Morigi *et al.*, 2014 (73)	Kidney	Acute ischemia-reperfusion and acute tubular necrosis
Wang *et al.*, 2018 (74)	Hepatic	Liver fibrosis
Maraldi *et al.*, 2013 (75)	Bone and cartilage	Extensive bone defects disease
Chang *et al.*, 2018 (76)	Ovarian	Ovarian dystrophy and fertility
Gosemann *et al* ., 2012 (77)	Inflammatory and autoimmune diseases	Graft-vs-host disease, inflammatory bowel disease, experimental autoimmune encephalomyelitis and systemic lupus erythematosus

Differentiation potential of human amniotic epithelial stem cells

Data from: https://www.ncbi.nlm.nih.gov/pmc/articles/PMC9596929/

"Amniotic fluid is the perfect regenerative fluid mixture and the perfect regenerative medicine treatment because it's the biologically ideal mixture of components to support tissue growth and regeneration." – Will Bozeman.

Yep, I just quoted myself, but it's a true statement and I've been saying that for a decade now. The balance of growth factors and proteins is literally arranged in perfect ratios, so ultimately it would be the perfect fluid to use, no lab alteration required.

In fact, my most popular and successful product ever produced was the simplest version: pure amniotic fluid. We didn't alter it in any way; we simply filtered it for safety and left the concentrations exactly as is. This was the most successful regenerative product I've ever created in one of my biotech companies.

PRP (PRFM, A2M, platelet lysate, and other PRP isolates): Immediately I want to say that PRP is not all the same, and what your doctor calls PRP in their office may be vastly different from PRP in another office under different processing techniques. Dosing and concentration are everything when it comes to PRP. Keep that in mind as I explain the basics here.

Platelet-derived growth factor (PDGF)	Enhances collagen synthesis, proliferation of bone cells, fibroblast chemotaxis and proliferative activity, macrophage activation
Transforming growth factor ß (TGF-ß)	Enhances synthesis of type I collagen, promotes angiogenesis, stimulates chemotaxis of immune cells, inhibits osteoclast formation and bone resorption
Vascular endothelial growth factor (VEGF)	Stimulates angiogenesis, migration and mitosis of endothelial cells, increases permeability of the vessels, stimulates chemotaxis of macrophages and neutrophils
Epidermal growth factor (EGF)	Stimulates cellular proliferation, differentiation of epithelial cells, promotes cytokine secretion by mesenchymal and epithelial cells
Insulin-like growth factor (IGF)	Promotes cell growth, differentiation, recruitment in bone, blood vessel, skin and other tissues, stimulates collagen synthesis together with PDGF
Fibroblast growth factor (FGF)	Promotes proliferation of mesenchymal cells, chondrocytes and osteoblasts, stimulates the growth and differentiation of chondrocytes and osteoblasts

Growth factors in PRP

Data from: https://www.ncbi.nlm.nih.gov/pmc/articles/PMC8046674/

Platelet-rich plasma was all the rage a couple of decades ago when a few high-end athletes mentioned getting PRP treatments for rapid recovery, which sparked a huge demand for PRP in the MSK field. Then a few celebrities and influencers promoted PRP for facials and hair regeneration, and then suddenly it was all the rage in esthetics – and still is. PRP is created by drawing your blood, spinning it down and concentrating the plasma, drawing that back out, and then reinjecting it into the damaged tissue.

So, with all the processing techniques and processes out there, we can isolate almost any particular element out of your plasma and reinject that particular element instead of the whole plasma concoction.

This is an excellent advancement in regenerative medicine because all the studies show that different isolates of PRP are great at doing different things. So yeah, it can get complicated, and I won't go too far into the weeds on this, but I'll briefly mention the ones listed in the heading of this section.

PRP is platelet-rich plasma and is simply concentrated plasma. PRFM is platelet-rich fibrin matrix, which is simply PRP with a slightly different processing technique to make the mixture react differently and maybe more useful in some scenarios.

A2M is alpha-2-macroglobulin and is great at inhibiting cartilage deterioration (which occurs in patients with osteoarthritis) by binding up the reactive proteins in your joints that cause cartilage deterioration.

Platelet lysate is one of the many isolates of PRP that can create enhanced healing effects on specific tissues. Again, the dosage is everything with each of these versions of PRP. Yeah, it gets complicated and there is a lot of research going into these various treatments. It's actively being proven that the concentrations of these treatments are just as important as what's in them.

In some studies, a 4x concentration of PRP does nearly nothing, while a 7x concentration crosses the threshold into tissue activity, all with the same stuff, just more concentrated. So don't worry too much about the particulars at the moment, but know that when a doctor says "PRP," you want to know what exactly it is they are talking about.

Exosomes or Secretomes: Exosomes are essentially the growth fluid used to grow stem cells in the lab. I create a plate of stem cells to grow in a dish and the nutrient-rich fluid the cells need is used by the cells and the leftover fluid has a lot of the beneficial elements of the stem cell growth process.

After the cells start growing, they produce little micro lipid packets of signaling proteins that are excreted from the cell, called exosomes – because they exit the cell – and they're little enclosed lipid bodies like bubbles, so "exit-body" or the more scientifically sounding "exosome" fits the description. They're also called secretomes because they're secreted from the cell.

Will's Industry Insight #12: "
A company reached out to me a year after exosomes were in the market wanting my help on distribution and growth with their new "unique amniotic fluid" product line.

I asked them a few questions because amniotic fluid was an official unique product designation, meaning it's not like anything else and the FDA recognizes this as a unique thing, which means you can't change it without calling it something else … meaning your brand of amniotic fluid can't be "unique amniotic fluid" and still be compliant.

They told me they were growing amniotic fluid in the lab. I asked how they were doing that because amniotic fluid doesn't grow in labs. They said they were culturing stem cells and taking the growth fluid and making amniotic fluid because they were using amniotic membrane stem cells and that's what amniotic fluid was, right? Simple logic … right? The fluid spins off from the amniotic membrane? You can see how complicated the definitions can be.

If stem cells are an apple orchard, exosomes are the truck loads of apples leaving the orchard.

The first lab to bring exosomes to market years ago was an associate of mine, and we chatted a few times about the possibility of using this product. My first thought was that it could be a really interesting category, but it wasn't even a market category at all, so how would it be viewed by regulators and the medical community? I didn't know at all. I told them it sounded interesting, but it would be an unknown risk to bring it to market.

Fast-forward a couple years and they were selling across the nation, and a dozen other groups were making their own exosome products. So, exosomes were all the hype for a few years and got a lot of negative attention, and, ultimately, you don't see them much anymore.

Exosomes are still around, but they got hammered by the FDA for misrepresentation because sales reps and companies were selling them under the wrong terms. They started out calling them stem cells like everything else, but when stem cells became a dirty word, they switched to calling exosomes "amniotic fluid." Why? Let me throw in a little Will's Industry Insight here to explain.

Keep in mind that I was on the phone with the top executives at this biotech company: the CEO, their Chief Medical Officer, their Chief Science Officer, and their Chief Sales Officer. They were the ones who were deciding how to educate their clients, doctors, on what this product was that they were selling.

I said, "What you're describing is not amniotic fluid, it's exosomes."

Long pause. "Yeah, we know it's actually exosomes, but," here are their own words and I wish I had recorded this, "it's too difficult to educate doctors on the nuances of different products, so we just call it amniotic fluid because they understand that and it's more acceptable to them."

So, there you have it: the reason for all the regulations and problems we've had in the regenerative medicine industry over the last five years. You can't call it what it isn't. So, after they got caught calling it the wrong thing, which I thoroughly warned them about, they were forced to change their description type to a new term, "amniotic derived fluid," which again, was all to avoid calling it what it actually was: exosomes.

All this was because it was too hard to explain exosomes and there were already major competitors in the market for exosomes and they wanted something unique that couldn't be replicated by competitors. So, this company thought they'd be clever and create a new market category, but the FDA moved all lab grown products into another classification later and that basically stopped everyone in their tracks on exosomes.

Peptides: This is an exciting new field of medicine with a lot of potential. Peptides are protein compound segments that are created to affect certain cellular responses. Stem cells are the orchard, exosomes are the apples, and peptides are the juice in the apples. Cells are looking for the signals from other cells to communicate and take action.

Peptides are great because they can be grown in the lab and all sorts of specific peptides can be isolated and grown in concentration. I believe there is exceptional biologic standardization potential with peptides, so I'm actively keeping an eye on peptides and looking forward to innovation in that field.

Prolotherapy: Prolotherapy is a dextrose sugar injection that agitates the tissues at the cellular level and creates a mild inflammation with a healing effect afterward, like doing an exfoliating scrub on your face to remove all the dead skin and the after-effect creates fine, smooth skin.

Some physicians wouldn't call prolotherapy a true regenerative medicine therapy in the same category as these other items above, but many do feel that it qualifies as a regenerative.

It's great of course, but you're not adding any regenerative elements to this process, you're simply agitating tissue to become mildly inflamed and then letting it heal back up. In short, it's simply creating a mild local tissue irritation through dextrose sugar crystals roughing up the cells and tissue and causing inflammation and mild tissue damage in that area for the cells to be agitated and triggered into healing.

I've talked to doctors who do consider it regenerative, but I've talked to a lot of doctors about this, and with all the better options out there, stem cells, PRP, and other options, it's hard to justify doing old-school prolotherapy except that it's so affordable because dextrose is really cheap, and the injections are very simple and easy.

That's the wrap-up on the general overview of regenerative medicine in the US. Keep in mind that by the time you read this, some of the things I mentioned may have new regulations and you may not find some of these options at all.

Now, let's talk about COPD and how regenerative medicine treatments are changing the entire treatment strategy for this condition. You have options, and stem cells for chronic respiratory conditions may be exactly what you need!

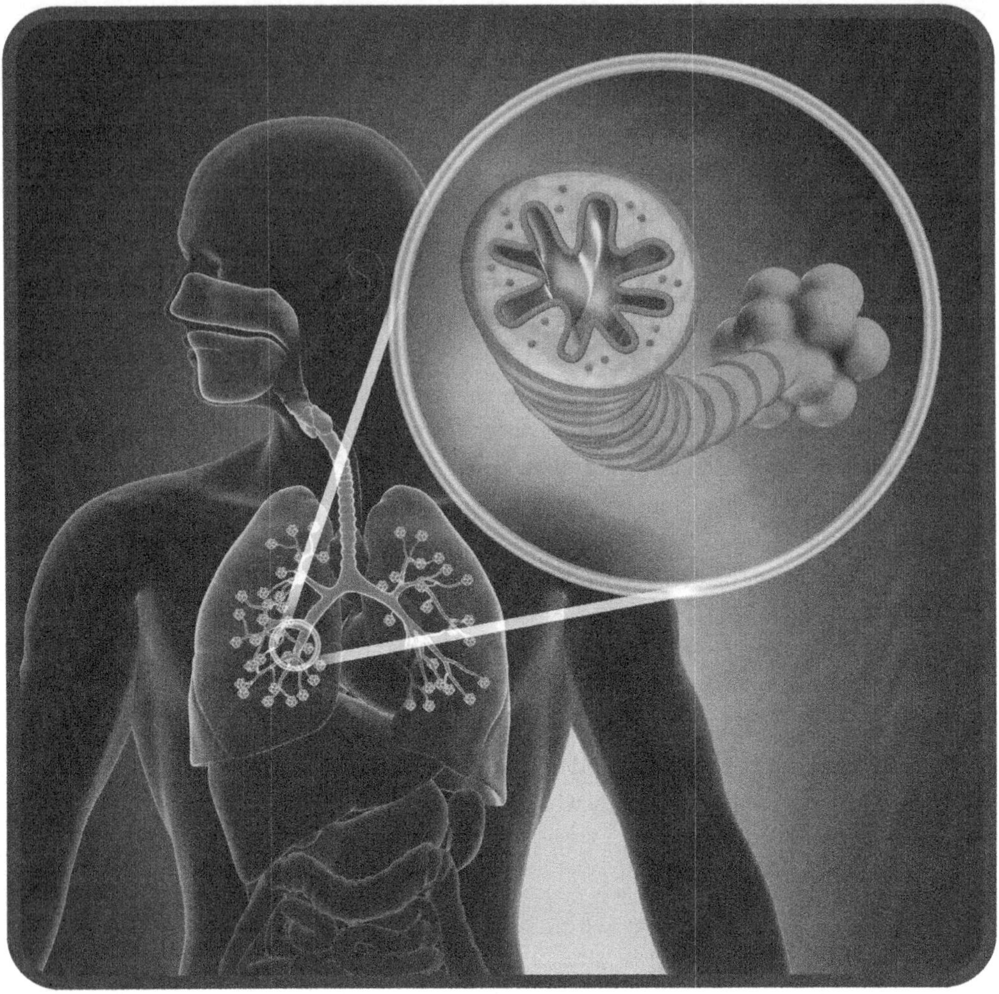

Chapter 3 - Introduction To COPD

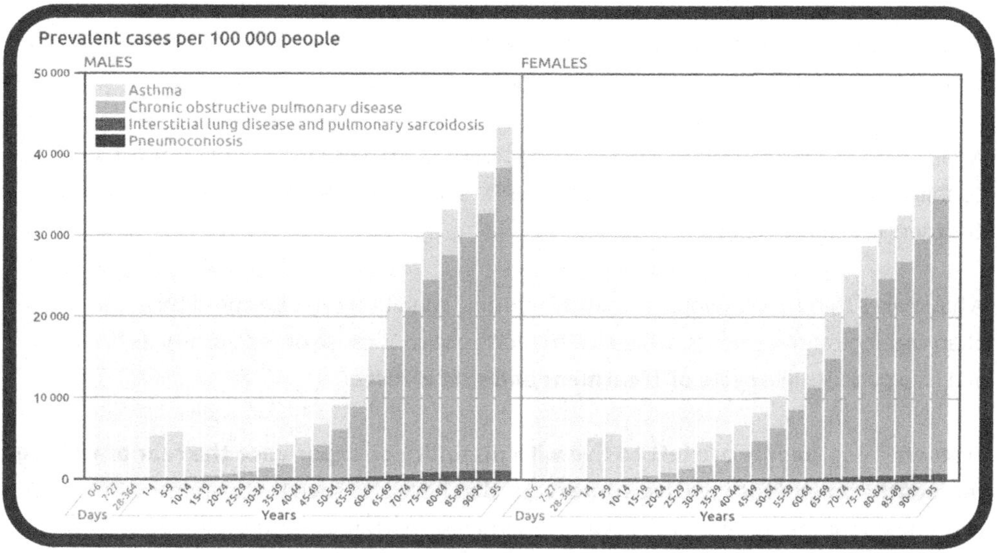

Global age-sex-specific prevalence of chronic respiratory diseases by disease category in 2017

Data from: https://www.ncbi.nlm.nih.gov/pmc/articles/PMC7284317/

Today, nearly 545 million people live with chronic respiratory conditions such as chronic obstructive pulmonary disease, or COPD. This figure represents a whopping 7.4% of the world's population, highlighting the severe burden of chronic respiratory diseases on the global healthcare system.

According to statistics from the European Union, diseases of the respiratory system are also responsible for 6.7 % of all deaths in the EU each year.

But to understand and address these respiratory conditions, it is important to look beyond the numbers. **Affecting the lungs and airways, chronic obstructive pulmonary disease makes it difficult to breathe and creates breathing-related problems**.

But this disease also creates a cascade of negative effects on an individual's health that go far beyond the respiratory system.

People with COPD may start to suffer from ongoing infections and chronic bronchitis, as well as complications like emphysema. The reduced airflow and oxygen circulation can, over time, deprive organs and tissues of essential nutrients, eventually leading to respiratory failure, heart failure, osteoporosis, sleep problems (and, consequently, daytime fatigue and declining cognitive health), and even dementia.

What's more, similarly to other chronic conditions, the exacerbation of discomfort and disability, can, in time, cause people with COPD to start experiencing mental health disorders like depression.

What makes things even worse is that this chronic condition can't be cured through pharmacological treatments, which fail to tackle the root cause of respiratory difficulties and trap patients in a **cycle of treatment and side effects**.

In severe cases, **people are left to live with disability or experience the fear of waiting for months on end for invasive surgery**. Studies have also seen that patients with COPD undergoing surgery have a higher risk of "morbidity, mortality, and duration of stay," making the prospect of surgery even more overwhelming.

This downward spiral is often **the starting point for a reduced health span (the number of years lived without disability) and shorter longevity,** as the body becomes increasingly vulnerable to secondary conditions.

The compromised immune system and reduced physical capacity make individuals more susceptible to other diseases, from infections to declining mental health, ultimately accelerating overall health decline.

But when it comes to restoring your health, it is important to keep in mind that most of the root causes of COPD stem from lifestyle choices and the environment rather than genetics. In turn, these **causes can be modified with the right proactive interventions**.

Stem cell therapy emerges as an innovative weapon in the battle against COPD. When combined with lifestyle modifications, **stem cell treatment harnesses the body's natural regenerative capabilities, offering a promising avenue for recovery**.

These cells can potentially repair damaged lung tissue and improve lung function, marking a shift towards innovative, restorative treatments.

Today, we know that COPD is making it harder to breathe for the over 16 million Americans who have been diagnosed with this disease. But there are also millions more people in the US and worldwide who see their lives and health status impacted by respiratory problems but have not yet been diagnosed. Fortunately, thanks to the availability of Lifestyle Medicine techniques and stem cell therapies, patients now have the chance to take their pulmonary health in their own hands and look at a brighter future.

Understanding This Respiratory Condition

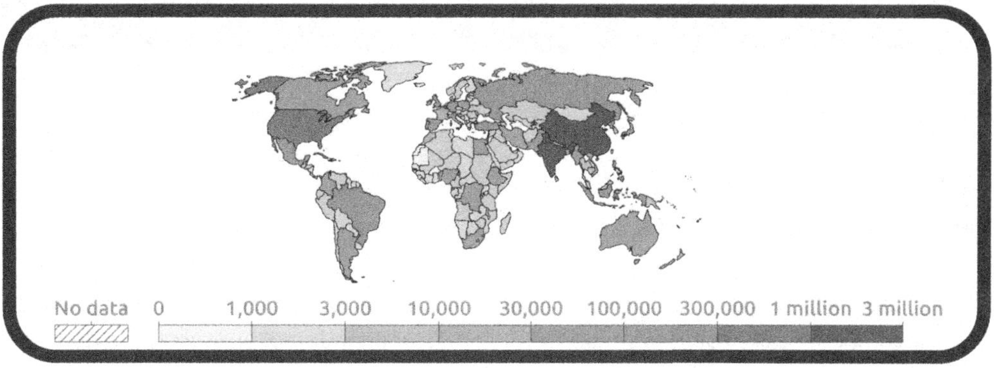

Deaths from Chronic Respiratory Diseases
Data from: https://ourworldindata.org/grapher/deaths-from-respiratory-disease

Chronic obstructive pulmonary disease is a term that describes a group of lung conditions characterized by chronic (long-term) airflow obstruction and significant breathing difficulties. In 2019, these chronic respiratory diseases were deemed to be the third-leading cause of death globally: they affected 455 million people and killed 4 million individuals worldwide.

An overview of the lung system

Your respiratory system, essentially your breathing apparatus, plays a pivotal role in keeping you alive. Think of it as a sophisticated air filter and gas exchange system. It starts with your nose or mouth, where air enters before traveling down your throat through the trachea. It then branches into two main tubes called bronchi.

These bronchi further divide into smaller tubes in the lungs known as bronchioles, ending in tiny air sacs called alveoli. Here's where the oxygen from the air you've inhaled passes into your bloodstream. Then, carbon dioxide, a waste product from your body, is expelled during exhalation.

But the respiratory system isn't just composed of physical structures. It is supported by the diaphragm, a strong muscle beneath your lungs that contracts and relaxes to pull air in and push it out. The several processes involved with respiration ensure that every cell in your body gets the oxygen it needs to function and removes carbon dioxide, a build-up of which could be dangerous.

Although, as you'll see below, this group of progressive respiratory diseases describes several health conditions, it primarily involves two main diseases: emphysema, where the air sacs of the lungs are damaged and stretched; and chronic bronchitis, characterized by inflammation and narrowing of the bronchial tubes, leading to mucus buildup.

These diseases may be caused by infection - but more commonly, they stem from exposure to toxic compounds like tobacco smoke (including secondhand smoke), asbestos, radon, and polluted air.

As they develop, these respiratory diseases limit airflow both in and out of the lungs, making every breath a challenge.

Today, the disease represents a critical concern for public health systems across the globe and significantly affects the lives and longevity of people around the world, both children and adults.

To understand how stem cells represent a non-invasive, non-pharmaceutical alternative to standard treatments for COPD, we'll first look at what you need to know about this disease, from its history to its symptoms and causes.

History Of COPD

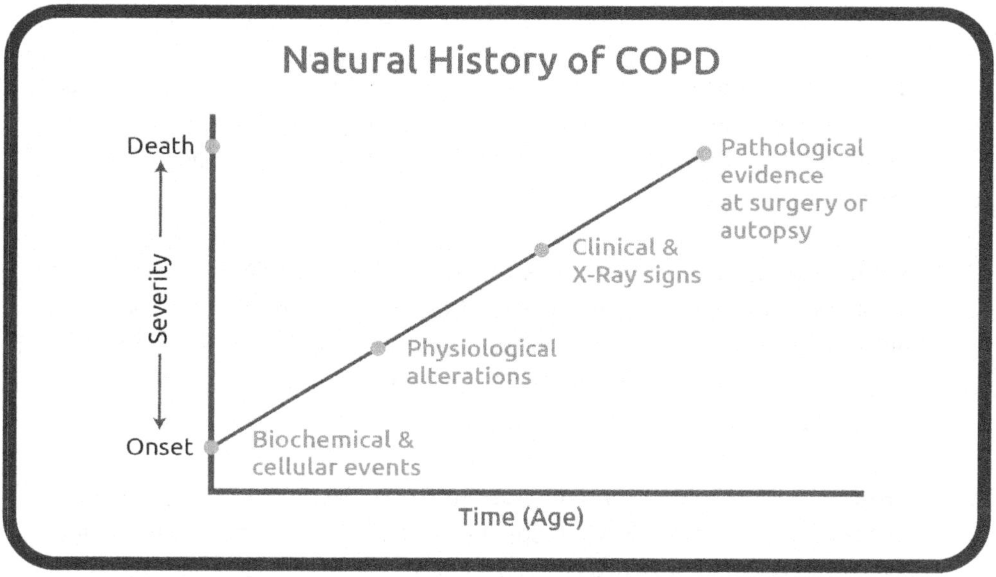

The Natural History of COPD
Data from: https://www.ncbi.nlm.nih.gov/pmc/articles/PMC2706597/figure/f3-copd-1-3/

Although people have suffered from lung conditions throughout history, initially, COPD was less about the disease itself and more about its symptoms: doctors had to deal with cases of airflow blockages, asthma-like symptoms, and pulmonary infections, but these were treated as standalone problems.

COPD gained recognition in the 18th century, when doctors began to piece together the respiratory difficulties they observed. However, it wasn't until the 20th century that COPD was identified as a specific disease. Some of the main milestones achieved by early research around this condition are:

- **1789:** Dr. Matthew Baillie published illustrations of emphysematous lungs, identifying emphysema as part of COPD pathology.

- **1814:** Charles Badham introduced the term "catarrh" for chronic cough and mucus secretion linked to bronchiolitis and chronic bronchitis, suggesting their role in COPD. A few years earlier, the same Badham had described acute and chronic bronchitis clearly for the first time.

- **1821:** Rene Laënnec, the inventor of the stethoscope, described emphysema in his Treatise on Chest Diseases, noting excessively inflated lungs that don't empty well and combining emphysema with chronic bronchitis in his descriptions. The different pulmonary diseases were categorized based on the different sounds they produced when listened to with the stethoscope.

- **1846:** John Hutchinson invented the spirometer, a pivotal tool in diagnosing COPD by measuring vital capacity. Vital capacity was defined as the maximum amount of air a person can forcibly exhale from the lungs after a maximum inhalation, a key measure for assessing respiratory health - and longevity.

- **1947:** Robert Tiffeneau and André Pinelli enhanced spirometry by introducing timed vital capacity, which allowed them to measure airflow and lung capacity, aiding in COPD diagnosis and therapeutic response assessment.

Since this research was published, the number of COPD cases has been on the rise. According to studies, the incidence of COPD increased by 85.89% from 1990 to 2019, and it is set to continue on this upward trend. There are several reasons behind this increase, including the aging of the population and the growing life expectancy.

However, there have also been some socioeconomic factors over the past decades that have made COPD a global health burden. These include:

- **Industrial revolution:** The introduction of coal-fired factories introduced massive amounts of smoke and soot into the air, significantly impacting lung health.
- **Cigarette smoke:** The widespread adoption of smoking in the 20th century sharply increased the prevalence of COPD, making it a leading cause of the disease today.
- **Use of asbestos:** Known for its durability, asbestos was a popular building material in the 1930s to the 1980s that, when inhaled, could lead to serious lung diseases, including COPD, lung cancer, mesothelioma, and asbestosis.
- **Air pollution:** The escalation of air pollution due to vehicle emissions and industrial activities contributes heavily to the incidence of COPD, especially in urban areas.
- **Urbanization.** Urban areas have rising population densities as well as higher levels of pollution, putting inhabitants at risk.

Vulnerability, Occurrence Levels, And Impact

Certain populations are more vulnerable to developing COPD than others. In the next chapters of this book, I'll talk more about the causes and risk factors of COPD.

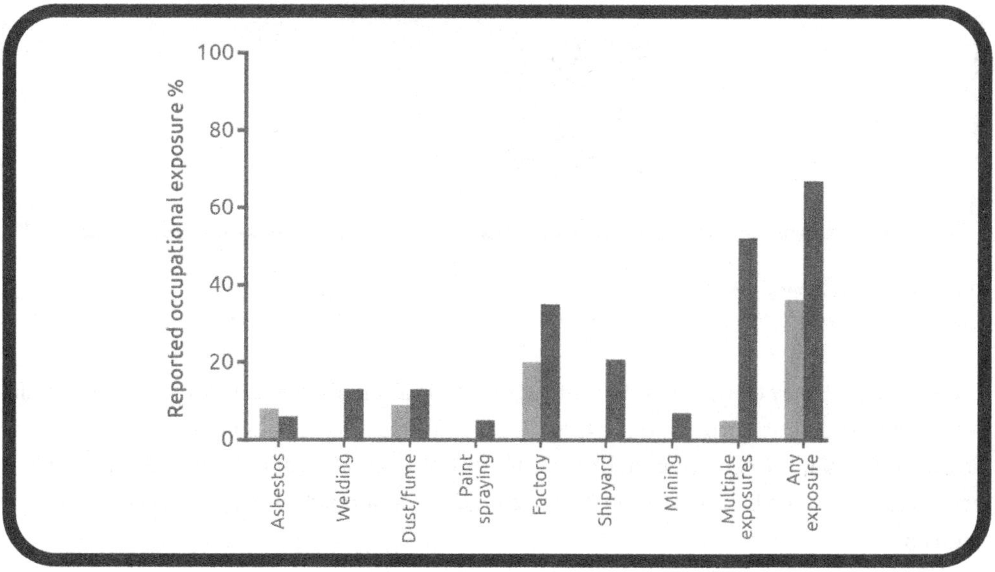

Specific occupational exposure in males and females.
Data from: https://erj.ersjournals.com/content/36/3/488

But to offer an overview, those at **greater risk of developing COPD include long-term smokers, individuals exposed to occupational hazards like dust and chemicals, and people living in areas with high air pollution.** Its occurrence has risen steadily, becoming the third leading cause of death worldwide.

In terms of the impact of this disease, the costs of care and economic burden on the healthcare system are just part of this multifaceted issue. The impact of **COPD extends beyond the individual, affecting families and the community as a whole due to its chronic, debilitating nature and the need for ongoing care.**

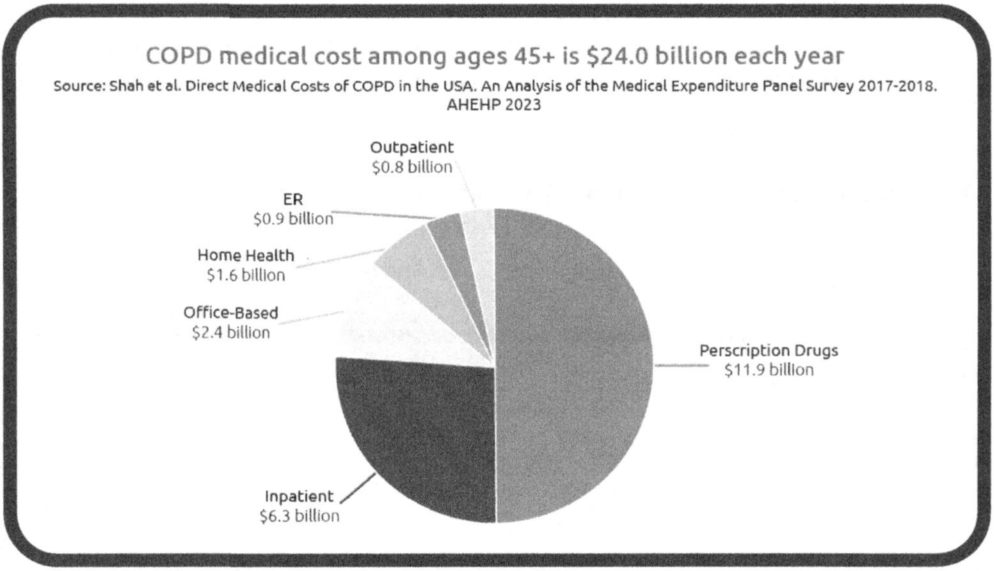

COPD Medical Cost Among Ages 45+
Data from: https://www.lung.org/research/trends-in-lung-disease/copd-trends-brief/copd-burden

Economically, it may lead to a significant burden on individuals due to lost productivity and high medical costs. According to the American Lung Association, patients with COPD spend an average of $4,322 each year on this condition. Between 2000 and 2018, COPD medical costs have increased by a whopping 72%, including an eightfold increase in prescription drug costs.

Future Considerations

Estimates suggest that the number of global cases could experience a 23% rise by 2025, which would equal over 600 million people affected by COPD. The increase is more likely to affect women, with cases expected to surge by 47.1% among female patients. Additionally, low- and middle-income regions will be the most affected.

Given these figures, it is clear that, moving forward, addressing COPD will require a multi-faceted approach that is not reactive nor based just on drugs or surgery. Not only is there an urgent need for enhanced research - but healthcare providers should pioneer prevention measures, patient resources, and innovative treatments.

Risk Factors And Possible Complications

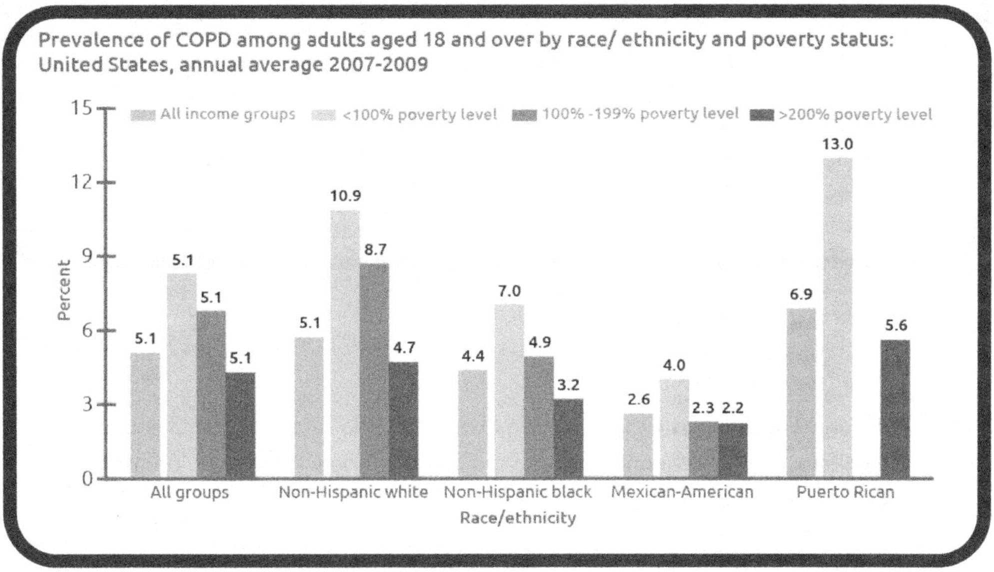

Data from: https://www.cdc.gov/nchs/products/databriefs/db63.htm

COPD can affect anyone, at any stage of life. However, it tends to be more common among women younger than 65. Adults with family income below the poverty level may also have a greater risk of developing this disease.

Other key risk factors of COPD include:

- **Smoking:** Smoking is the primary catalyst for COPD, with up to 90% of cases linked to cigarette smoke, with 20% of smokers expected to develop this disease at some point in life. This occurs because tobacco smoke releases over 7000 chemicals and damages the lungs, impairing their ability to function effectively.

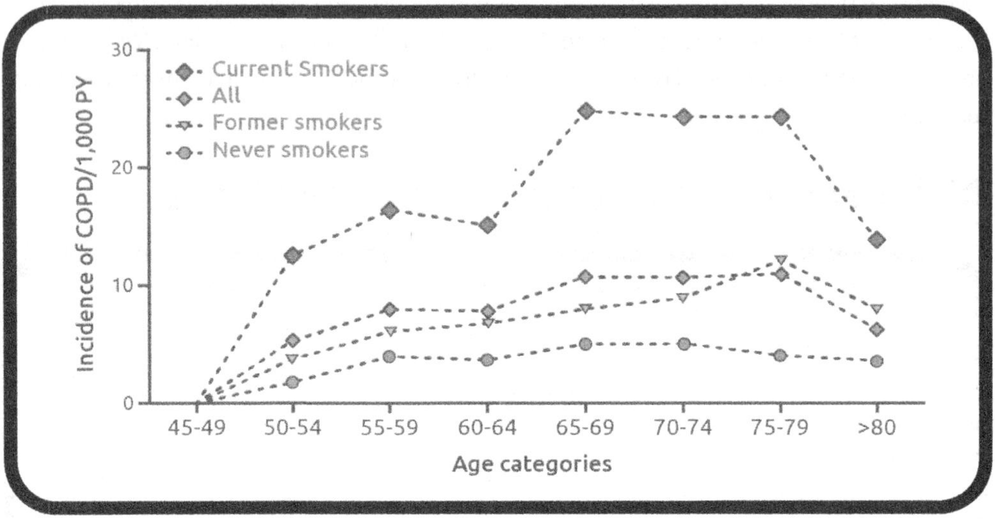

Age specific incidence of COPD by smoking behavior.

Data from: https://www.ncbi.nlm.nih.gov/pmc/articles/PMC5005388/

- **Environmental exposure:** Long-term exposure to harmful pollutants, such as industrial emissions, chemical fumes, and indoor air pollutants like biomass fuel used for cooking, accelerates lung damage.

- **Occupational hazards:** Jobs that involve dust, fumes, or toxic gasses put workers at a higher risk. Studies have pointed to professions such as construction, mining, and welding as being particularly vulnerable. It is estimated that occupational exposure contributes to an estimated 14% of all COPD cases and 31% of cases among never smokers. Some professions at risk include:

    - Coal miners
    - Construction workers
    - Welders
    - Textile workers
    - Agricultural workers
    - Firefighters

- Genetics: Alpha-1 antitrypsin (AAT) deficiency is a rare genetic condition that can predispose individuals to COPD. People with this condition don't make enough AAT, a protein created by the liver with the role of protecting the lungs. When the levels of AAT are too low, the lungs are unprotected and more prone to damage from smoking, toxins, and pollutants.

- Asthma: Individuals with a history of asthma are at a greater risk of developing COPD, as both conditions share a common pathway of airway obstruction and inflammation.

- Age and gender: Typically, COPD is diagnosed in people aged 40 and above, indicating that risk increases with age. Historically more common among men, the increasing rates of smoking among women have seen their vulnerability rise to match the levels seen among males.

Studies have also seen that the incidence can vary by ethnicity, with Caucasian individuals being the most affected.

Possible Complications

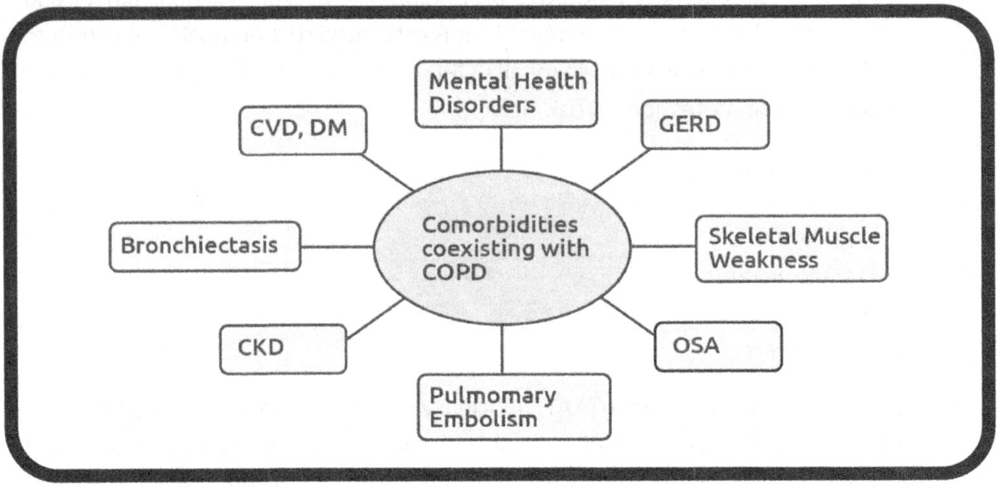

Clinical comorbidities coexisting with COPD

Data from: https://www.ncbi.nlm.nih.gov/pmc/articles/PMC10037643/

Left unaddressed, COPD's progression can lead to severe complications, impacting overall health and quality of life. Some of the most common complications among patients include:

- **Respiratory infections:** The damage to lung tissue makes it easier for infections to take hold, leading to increased vulnerability to colds, flu, and pneumonia. Being regularly ill or unwell can then impact mental well-being as well as employability, productivity, and interpersonal relationships.

- **Heart problems:** COPD can cause an increase in blood pressure within the arteries to the lungs (pulmonary hypertension). This can lead to a range of heart problems, and eventually, life-threatening conditions like heart failure.

- **Chronic bronchitis:** Chronic bronchitis, a complication of COPD, is characterized by inflammation of the bronchial tubes, leading to persistent cough and excessive mucus production. This condition can stem from a range of causes, but it often develops as a consequence of prolonged exposure to irritants that damage the airways and lungs, exacerbating respiratory difficulties in COPD patients.

- **Pneumothorax:** This condition refers to a potentially life-threatening buildup of air within the pleural cavity, which can cause the lungs to collapse. It occurs more frequently in people with lung diseases, including COPD, in individuals with tall, thin bodies, and in smokers.

- **Depression and anxiety:** Living with a chronic disease like COPD can lead to mental health issues, as coping with decreased lung function and reduced quality of life takes its toll on mental well-being. A study published in 2023 shows that the prevalence of depression is consistently elevated among those with COPD and that those with severe COPD are twice as likely to develop depression compared with patients with mild COPD.

For those diagnosed with COPD, management strategies focus on minimizing exposure to pollutants, quitting smoking, and, importantly, regular health check-ups to monitor lung function. For healthy individuals, prevention strategies such as environmental and lifestyle interventions can help safeguard respiratory health.

We'll look at these management and prevention strategies more in-depth in later chapters of this book. However, it is important to keep in mind that addressing respiratory health conditions early on is vital to **alter the course of the disease, reducing the risk of complications and offering a better prognosis and quality of life.**

Causes

COPD is a progressive condition that begins to manifest with mild symptoms, which get exponentially worse over time. The causes are multifaceted: in most cases, patients develop COPD as a result of a combination of environmental, lifestyle, and genetic factors.

Below, we'll look at the primary causes of COPD, as well as risk factors and contributors.

Primary Causes

- **Cigarette smoking.** One of the leading causes of COPD is cigarette smoking. The risk increases with the number of years and amount of tobacco smoked. This occurs because cigarette smoke is composed of a complex mixture of over 7,000 chemicals, including toxins such as tar, carbon monoxide, nitrogen oxides, and various volatile organic compounds.

When inhaled, these substances trigger a cascade of inflammatory responses in the respiratory tract. Here are some examples:

- Tar, a particulate matter, coats the lung tissue, impairing the function of cilia (hairlike vibrating structures found on the surface of certain cells) and leading to mucus overproduction.
- Carbon monoxide binds to hemoglobin more effectively than oxygen, significantly reducing oxygen delivery to tissues.
- Nitrogen oxides (and other oxidizing agents) damage lung tissue directly, leading to emphysema.

The chronic inflammation caused by chemicals and toxins contributes to the thickening and narrowing of the airways. At the same time, malfunctioning of the alveolar walls (collagen and elastic fibers that support the expansion and contraction of the lungs) reduces the surface area available for gas exchange.

The combination of these effects culminates in reduced lung function, which is synonymous with COPD. Studies estimate that the prevalence of COPD in never smokers is close to 6.5% while in ever smokers (even those who quit) can be as high as 17.8%.

- **Environmental exposure to toxins.** Long-term exposure to lung irritants may play a critical role in the development of COPD. These irritants and toxins include:

    - Air pollution: Both indoor and outdoor air pollutants (airborne particulate matter [or PM2.5] and ozone) contribute to COPD. Indoor pollution has been identified as the leading cause of COPD in women. This disease, which can arise due to indoor cooking with biomass fuels in poorly ventilated spaces, is a major issue in developing countries.
    - Occupational dust and chemicals: Inhaling dust, fumes, and chemicals in the workplace can damage the lungs. Industries such as mining, construction, and manufacturing are particularly at risk.
    - Secondhand smoke exposure: Regular inhalation of tobacco smoke emitted by others can also damage the lungs over time, leading to COPD.

- **Genetic causes.** Although most cases of COPD derive from a combination of lifestyle and environmental factors, there may be some genetic contributors to be aware of. These include alpha-1 antitrypsin deficiency (AATD).

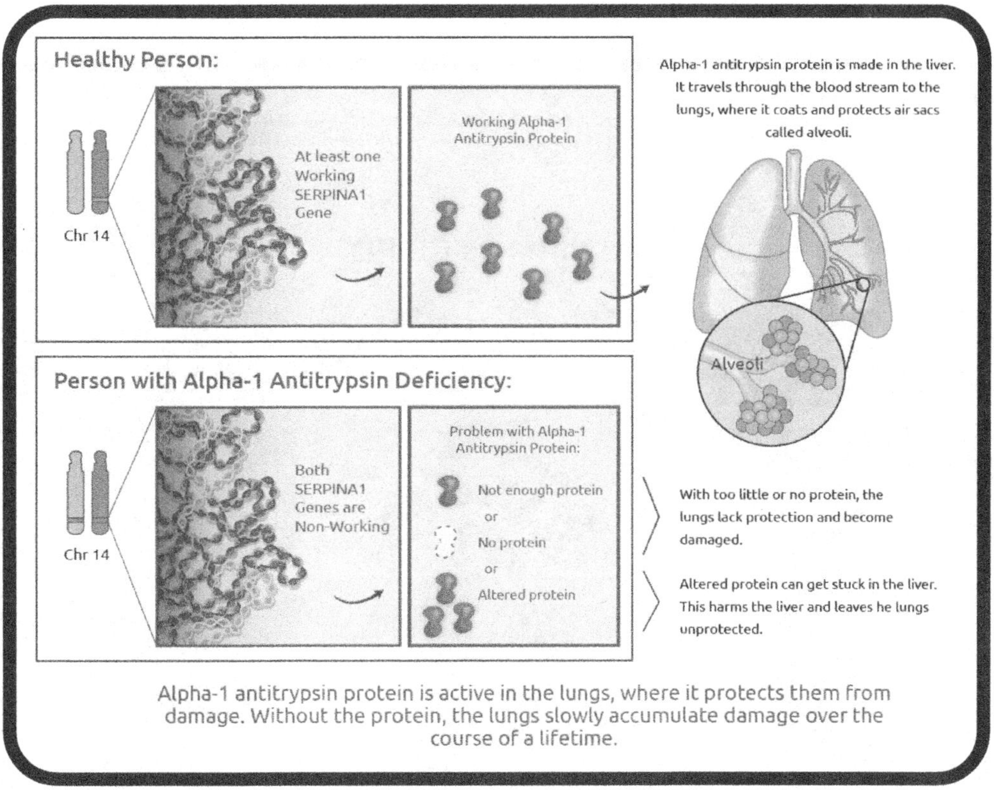

Alpha-1 antitrypsin protein is active in the lungs, where it protects them from damage. Without the protein, the lungs slowly accumulate damage over the course of a lifetime.

Data from: https://learn.genetics.utah.edu/content/genetics/alpha1/

As we've seen above, this is a genetic disorder that results in lower levels of alpha-1 antitrypsin (AAT) protein, which protects the lungs from neutrophil elastase. When AAT levels are too low, lung tissue can be easily damaged, leading to COPD even in nonsmokers.

Other Contributors

- **Asthma:** Chronic asthma can lead to changes in lung function and inflammation, which are the same changes seen in COPD. The risk of COPD is higher when asthmatic individuals also have a smoking habit.

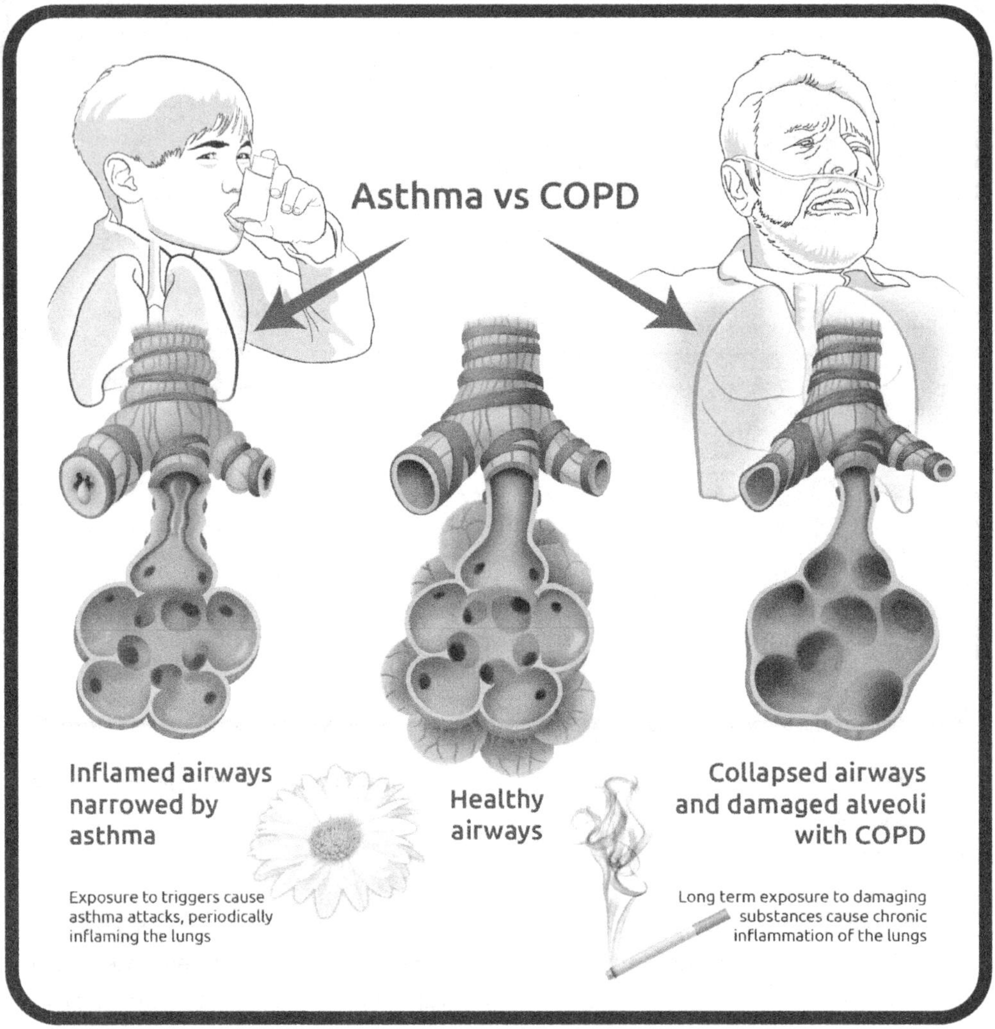

Asthma Vs COPD

Data from: https://www.buoyhealth.com/learn/asthma-vs-copd#overview

Asthma vs COPD: What are the differences?

Asthma is a reversible respiratory condition characterized by airway inflammation, leading to temporary narrowing of the airways, which can improve with medication or over time. COPD, on the other hand, is characterized by irreversible damage to the lungs and airways, primarily caused by long-term exposure to irritants, leading to permanent airflow limitation.

While both conditions present with symptoms like wheezing and shortness of breath, asthma typically manifests in early life, whereas COPD is more common in older adults with a history of smoking or exposure to pollutants.

- **Respiratory infections:** Frequent severe respiratory infections during childhood can impair lung growth, increasing the risk of developing COPD later in life.

Why Understanding The Causes Of COPD Is Important

The pathogenesis (the development of the disease) of COPD involves inflammation and structural changes in the lungs. For example, irritant exposure causes the airways and air sacs to lose their elastic quality.

Over time, the walls between many of the air sacs are destroyed and the walls of the airways become thickened, causing the airways to become clogged with mucus and unable to expand. Collectively, these changes restrict airflow and reduce the ability of the lungs to conduct gas exchange efficiently.

These changes are dramatic, but not immediately visible from the outside. Because of this, it is important to have a thorough understanding of how your lifestyle choices impact your lung health and risk of COPD. This is even more true for people who have a genetic predisposition or have asthma, so that the risk can be handled effectively.

While COPD remains incurable, recognizing and mitigating these causative factors can play a significant role in prevention and management, significantly improving the quality of life for those affected.

Symptoms

As I have shown above, the development of COPD may not happen overnight, and the early signs are easy to overlook. However, if left untreated, the symptoms often worsen over time and become disabling or life-threatening.

Because of this, recognizing these signs and symptoms early on can be pivotal in managing the disease's progression and improving the quality of life for those affected. In the sections below, we'll look at the major symptoms of COPD, as well as the telltale signs you should be aware of.

In any case, if you suspect that your respiratory health is threatened or you've noticed changes in your lung capacity (e.g.: you often find yourself out of breath) you should not delay in getting a comprehensive diagnosis.

Major Symptoms

Below are some of the symptoms that characterize COPD. You'll notice that several of these can easily be mistaken for the symptoms of other respiratory conditions, including asthma and chest infections.

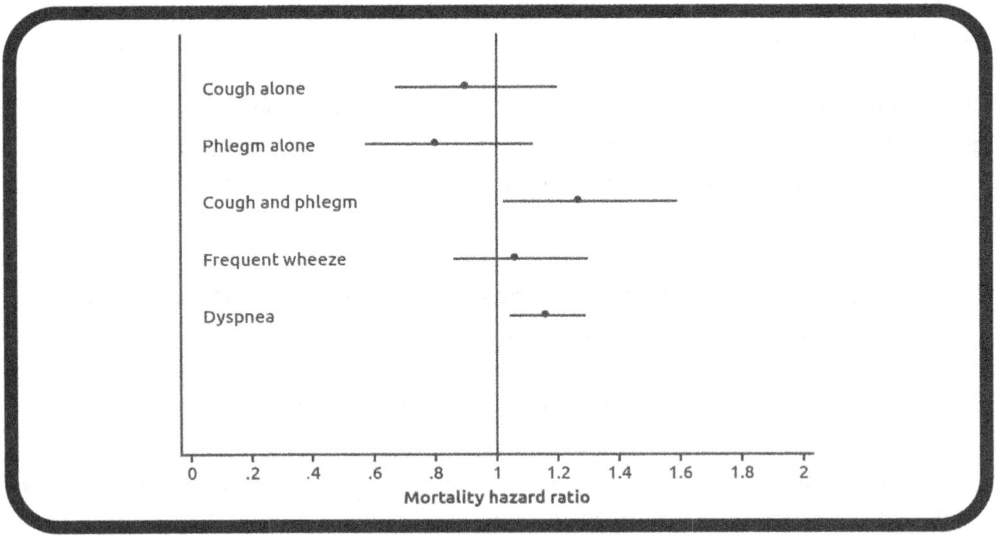

Associations between individual symptoms and mortality over 12 years.

Data from: https://www.ncbi.nlm.nih.gov/pmc/articles/PMC5120399/

- **Persistent cough:** Often referred to as a "smoker's cough," this can be the first indicator of COPD. The cough is usually more pronounced in the morning and produces a significant amount of mucus (known as "productive" cough). Smoker's cough in COPD becomes chronic and has been seen to be associated with early development of this disease and mortality.

- **Shortness of breath:** Initially, this may only occur with exertion but can become more persistent as the disease progresses. In individuals with COPD, shortness of breath occurs due to narrowed airways and damaged lung tissue, which significantly interfere with airflow and reduce the lungs' capacity to take in oxygen and get rid of carbon dioxide.

  This inhibited airflow and impaired gas exchange lead to increased effort to breathe, which manifests as breathlessness, especially during physical activity. However, over time, you may begin to feel breathlessness even when at rest.

- **Frequent respiratory infections:** Individuals with COPD are more susceptible to colds, flu, and pneumonia, which can exacerbate symptoms and lead to further lung damage.

  Let's look at pneumonia, for example. Pneumonia is an infection in one or both lungs caused by bacteria, viruses, or fungi, leading to inflammation and the filling of air sacs with fluid or pus. This infection can damage the lungs' alveoli (air sacs) and impair the exchange of oxygen and carbon dioxide, sometimes resulting in scarring or fibrosis.

  Such scarring can lead to long-lasting lung damage by reducing the lungs' elasticity and function, making it harder to breathe and properly oxygenate the blood. Because of these changes in the lungs, COPD and pneumonia are often comorbidities.

- **Wheezing:** Wheezing occurs as air struggles to pass through constricted or obstructed airways, a common symptom in conditions like asthma and COPD. This whistling sound, most noticeable during exhalation, is caused by the vibration of narrowed air passages as they try to accommodate the flow of air.

- **Chest tightness:** This sensation results from the difficulty in moving air through the airways, which become inflamed and narrowed in respiratory conditions. The muscles around the chest may also tighten in an attempt to facilitate breathing, especially during physical exertion or exposure to cold air, exacerbating the feeling of tightness. This symptom is worsened by physical activity or cold temperatures.

- **Increased mucus production:** In response to irritation or inflammation of the airways, the body's defense mechanism triggers an increased production of mucus, which has the role of trapping and eliminating pathogens or particles. However, this excessive mucus can accumulate, clogging the airways and making it more difficult to breathe, often triggering a cough - which is the body's attempt to clear blockages.

Other Indicators

The symptoms above are clear indicators that you may have a respiratory condition. In some cases, you'll need to obtain a comprehensive diagnosis to determine whether more generic symptoms such as persistent cough or chest tightness indicate COPD or another condition.

You may also experience other signs and symptoms that are non-specific, but they can help doctors create a comprehensive clinical picture of what's affecting your lungs. These include:

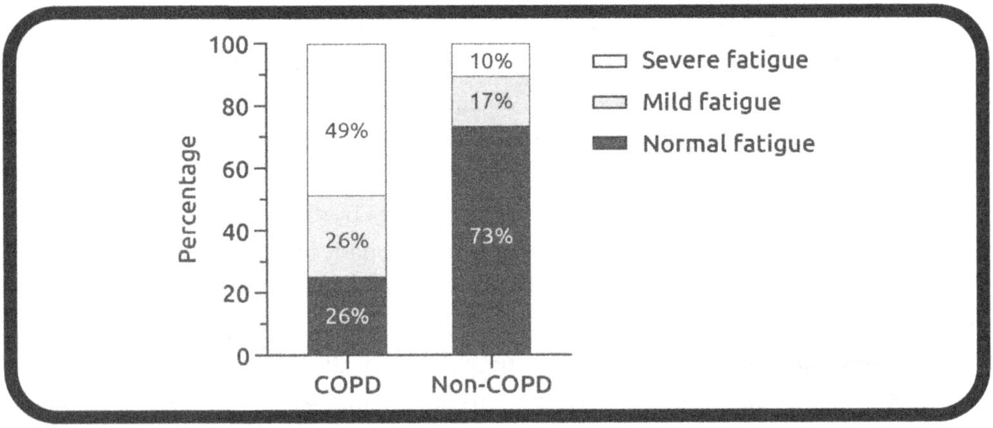

Associations between individual symptoms and mortality over 12 years.

Data from: https://www.ncbi.nlm.nih.gov/pmc/articles/PMC5120399/

- **Fatigue:** As the body works harder to breathe, COPD can lead to a significant loss of energy, making daily activities more challenging. Studies show that chronic fatigue is highly prevalent in patients with COPD compared to healthy individuals.
- **Weight loss:** Advanced stages of COPD can lead to weight loss and muscle wastage, partly due to the increased energy expenditure from the effort of breathing.
- **Swelling of the ankles, feet, or legs:** The reduced ability to exercise can cause fluid to build up in the body, leading to peripheral edema.
- **Cyanosis:** A bluish tint to the lips or fingernail beds (cyanosis) may appear when your COPD worsens. This sign indicates lower oxygen levels in the blood and requires immediate medical attention.

How Symptoms Develop In COPD

Symptoms of COPD typically develop slowly and can be easy to overlook in the early stages.

Many people mistake their early symptoms for a normal part of aging or a result of their smoking habits.

However, as the disease progresses, symptoms become more severe and interfere with daily tasks. If left untreated, these symptoms can permanently impair respiratory health and lead to disability or early mortality.

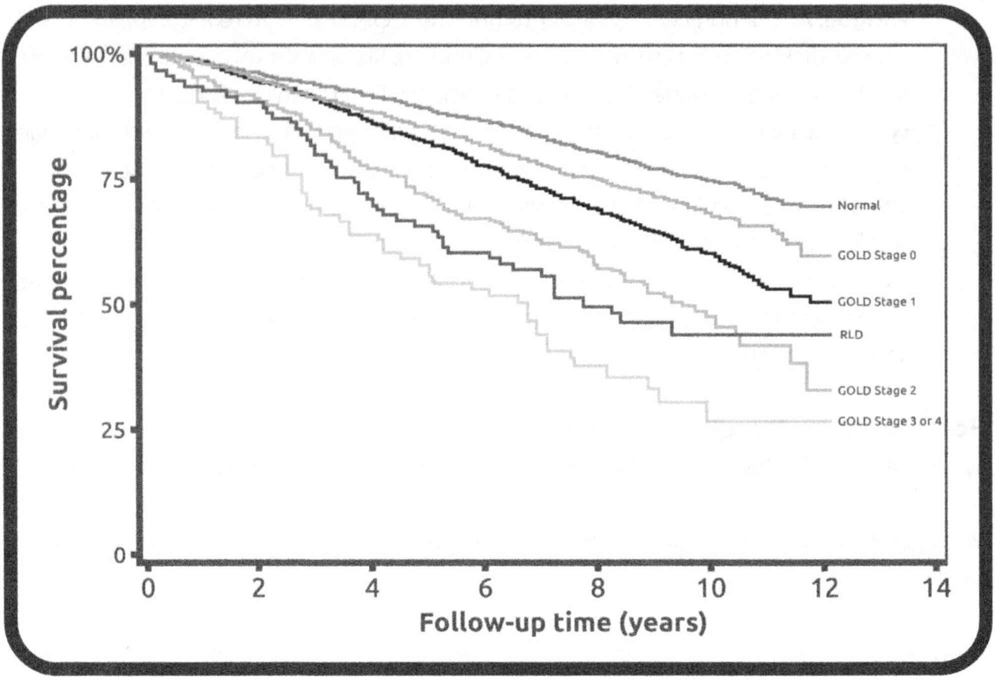

Kaplan–Meier survival curves of all 6,261 participants age 50 and over in NHANES III, stratified by lung function impairment

Data from: https://www.ncbi.nlm.nih.gov/pmc/articles/PMC2672796/figure/f2-copd-4-137/

Studies have shown that, in never smokers, COPD only mildly affects life expectancy. However, in smokers, COPD can significantly reduce life expectancy, according to the disease stage.

Here's an overview of life reduction for a male with COPD aged 65 (these figures are in addition to the 3.5 years lost due to smoking):

- Stage 1 - 0.3 years
- Stage 2 - 2.2 years
- Stage 3 or 4 - 5.8 years

Although the symptoms of COPD worsen over the course of many years, sometimes a sudden worsening of symptoms can occur. This is known as "COPD exacerbation," an event often triggered by an infection or another health problem. These exacerbations can significantly impact an individual's health status suddenly and without warning.

In both cases, recognizing the symptoms of COPD and seeking an accurate diagnosis can help you slow the progression of the disease, manage symptoms effectively, and maintain an active lifestyle for as long as possible.

Chapter 3 - Takeaways

- COPD is a leading cause of death worldwide. It is a disease characterized by chronic airflow obstruction and breathing difficulties. This disease involves several diseases, but mainly emphysema and chronic bronchitis.
- Key causes of COPD include smoking, environmental pollutants, occupational hazards, and genetic predispositions.
- Historical perspectives show COPD recognition evolved from understanding symptoms to identifying the disease in the 20th century.
- Socioeconomic factors, such as the Industrial Revolution, widespread smoking, and air pollution, have contributed to the rise in COPD cases.
- Risk factors for developing COPD include long-term smoking, exposure to pollutants, certain occupations, and genetics.
- Complications of COPD can be severe, affecting not only respiratory health but also leading to heart problems, infections, and mental health issues.
- Recognizing and understanding the primary causes of COPD - from cigarette smoking to genetic factors - are key to prevention and management.
- Symptoms of COPD, such as persistent cough, shortness of breath, and wheezing, develop slowly and worsen over time, highlighting the importance of early detection.
- COPD management strategies focus on minimizing pollutant exposure, smoking cessation, and regular health check-ups.

Chapter 4 - Physical Findings On Patients With COPD

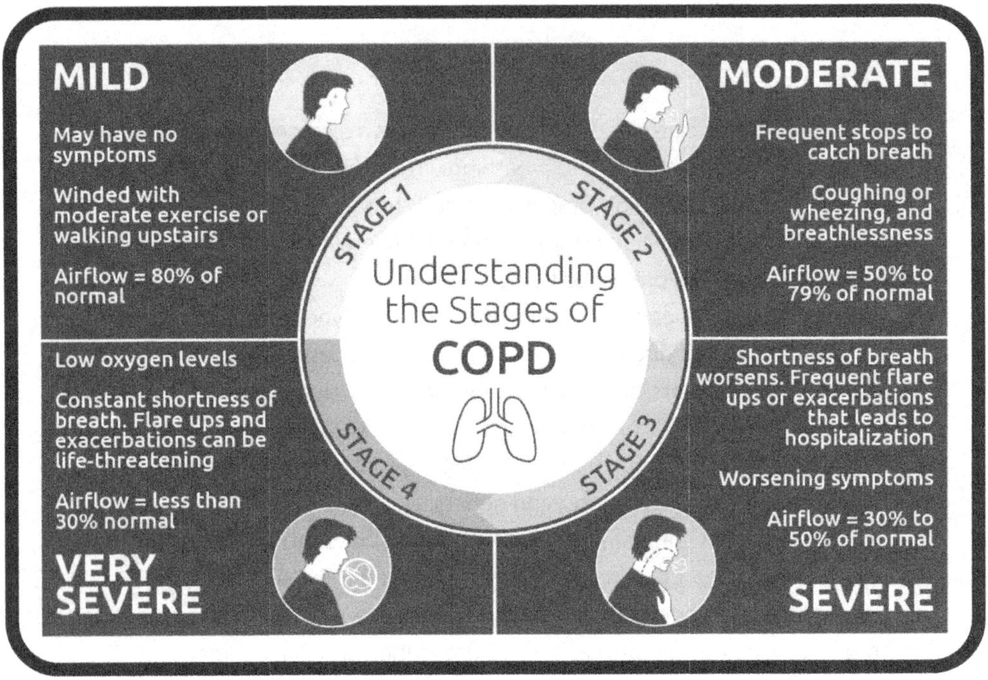

Stages of COPD

Data from: https://www.templehealth.org/services/conditions/chronic-obstructive-pulmonary-disease-copd

Chronic obstructive pulmonary disease manifests in the body in several distinct ways with both specific and non-specific symptoms. These signs can be observed through careful physical examination, which makes an accurate evaluation and diagnosis carried out by an expert a critical starting point for managing the disease.

As we have seen above, COPD primarily affects the lungs, but its physical manifestations can be extended to several other systems, organs, and tissues in the body. Afterall, oxygen is the most important element in our metabolism process and any illness that diminishes oxygen capacity directly impacts the rest of our body and systems.

Let's start with **the "hallmark" of COPD: the limitation of airflow**, a consequence of chronic inflammation in the airways and the destruction of lung tissue. Over time, these pathological changes lead to physical signs that a skilled clinician can identify during a physical examination.

COPD is categorized in stages by the GOLD standard, which stands for: "Global Initiative for Chronic Obstructive Lung Disease," an initiative started by the National Heart, Lung, and Blood Institute, National Institutes of Health, and the World Health Organization in 1997.

Each stage has different associated symptoms and likely complications and is based on several factors, including symptom severity, acceleration of disease, frequency of hospitalization due to COPD, and results from spirometry tests (a test that checks the amount and speed of air as you exhale).

The stages of COPD as per the GOLD standard are:

- **Stage 1:** mild COPD - In mild COPD, an individual may have a chronic cough. At this stage, lung function begins to decline but might not be noticeable to the person, because the airway flow is still at or above 80% of the expected value. You may not even experience breathlessness or only during significant physical exertion.

- **Stage 2:** moderate COPD - During this stage, symptoms become more noticeable. Individuals may experience increased breathlessness during physical activities, continued coughing, and increased sputum production (expectoration). Lung function further decreases, with airway flow ranging between 50% and 79% of the expected value. This is often the stage where individuals seek medical advice.

- **Stage 3:** severe COPD - Breathlessness becomes more marked at this stage, significantly affecting quality of life. Individuals may struggle with everyday tasks and suffer from frequent exacerbations (sudden worsening of symptoms). Lung function drops to between 30% and 49% of the predicted value. Patients at this stage may require significant medical intervention and the use of long-term oxygen therapy.

- **Stage 4:** very severe or end-stage COPD - This stage is marked by very limited lung function, airway flow less than 30% of the expected value, and chronic respiratory failure. These symptoms make this stage potentially life-threatening. Symptoms at this stage are severe, with individuals experiencing significant breathlessness even when they are at rest. Exacerbations that occur during this stage can be life-threatening, and patients may rely on extensive oxygen therapy and medication regimen, and surgical intervention becomes critical for managing the disease.

Understanding the signs associated with COPD is essential for anyone involved in the care of patients with COPD, from pulmonologists to primary care providers and beyond. It is also important for the patient to understand what the manifestations of COPD are.

Especially in subjects at risk or smokers, being aware of what COPD looks like can lead to early diagnosis and management.

Here are, in depth, the findings through which COPD manifests.

General Findings

COPD presents a range of physical signs. These tend to evolve over time, usually years, from early indicators to more severe systemic manifestations. Initially, the signs of COPD might be easily overlooked or attributed to aging, smoking, or a sedentary lifestyle.

However, as these signs get worse, both patients and healthcare providers can begin to create a comprehensive clinical picture that is likely to point to COPD. **COPD is a chronic and systemic disease, affecting not only the lungs but multiple organs and systems.**

Before diving into the different manifestations of this condition, let's look at what to expect at the different stages of the disease:

- **Early signs:** In the early stages, individuals may experience persistent cough, sputum production, and a mild - and, yet, progressive - difficulty in breathing, especially during physical activities.

  These symptoms stem from the inflammation and narrowing of the airways, combined with the destruction of lung tissue, characteristic of COPD.

- **Respiratory involvement:** The primary organ system affected by COPD is, undoubtedly, the respiratory system. Chronic exposure to irritants leads to an inflammatory response in the lung tissue.

  In turn, this leads to airflow limitation, hyperinflation (the abnormal increase in the size of air spaces within the lungs), and a decrease in gas exchange efficiency. This can manifest as shortness of breath, wheezing, and a chronic cough.

- **Systemic manifestations:** If COPD is left unmanaged, you are likely to experience more widespread - or systemic - effects:

  - A marked decline in physical stamina and endurance, making everyday activities increasingly challenging.

  - Unintended weight loss and muscle wasting due to decreased oxygen supply and increased energy expenditure from labored breathing.

  - An increase in anxiety and depression rates, likely linked to chronic illness and decreased quality of life.

  - Sleep quality may deteriorate due to nocturnal symptoms and oxygen desaturation (when the level of oxygen in the blood falls below the normal range), leading to fatigue and daytime sleepiness.

  - Emerging evidence suggests that chronic hypoxemia may impact cognitive functions, including memory, learning, processing speed and function, and concentration, potentially due to reduced oxygen supply to the brain.

When COPD progresses, patients begin to experience frequent exacerbations and exponentially worse symptoms. This causes a compounded effect that rapidly deteriorates an individual's quality of life, making comprehensive and prompt COPD management critical.

Skin

The skin, being the largest organ of the body, often mirrors the internal health of an individual, and it is one of the first affected by the systemic effects of COPD.

The **manifestations of COPD in the skin are primarily due to the chronic, systemic inflammation and the decreased oxygenation associated with the disease.** Reduced oxygen levels can lead to changes in skin color and texture.

These are some of the first outwardly visible signs of COPD and, by reflecting the severity of COPD, they offer visual cues about the patient's respiratory health.

Here are some of the skin symptoms to watch out for:

- **Cyanosis.** This is a bluish discoloration of the skin, especially evident in the lips, fingertips, and toes. This occurs due to insufficient oxygenation of the blood or low levels of oxygen in the blood. This is a common complication in advanced stages of COPD, where the lungs and respiratory system are malfunctioning and are unable to support efficient gas exchange, leading to decreased arterial oxygen levels.

- **Peripheral edema.** While not a skin condition per se, this symptom described the swelling of the lower extremities, usually in the ankles and feet, especially in the later stages of the disease. This swelling, which occurs due to the abnormal build-up of fluids, can cause significant changes in the skin, including tightness and increased risk of wounds.

Peripheral edema: a warning sign of cor pulmonale?

Edema may indicate cor pulmonale, a potentially life-threatening condition characterized by the enlargement and failure of the right side of the heart. This enlargement stems from excessively high blood pressure in the pulmonary arteries (pulmonary hypertension).

This condition often stems from COPD or other lung disorders that affect breathing. This is because, in these disorders, inflammation and constriction of the airways, along with damage to the lung tissue, obstruct airflow, making it difficult for air to move in and out of the lungs. This impeded airflow causes a decrease in oxygen levels and an increase in carbon dioxide in the blood. This imbalance prompts the pulmonary arteries to constrict - and when they contract, the blood pressure within them increases. This high pressure can cause life-threatening complications like edema and cor pulmonale.

- **Clubbing.** Clubbing describes the bulbous enlargement of the ends of fingers or toes, a symptom that is often accompanied by changes in the angle between the nails and nail beds. Clubbing is a sign of chronic hypoxemia, and in the context of COPD, it suggests a persistent and life-threatening reduction in oxygen levels.

- **Venous stasis.** This condition involves changes in the skin of the legs due to poor circulation. It can lead to discoloration, thickening, and ulcers.

  In patients with COPD, venous stasis occurs due to the inhibited venous return (the blood flow back to the heart) from the lower extremities, which occurs due to the reduced cardiac output and elevated pressure in the pulmonary circuit (the pathway blood takes between heart and lungs for oxygen exchange).

Upper And Lower Extremities

COPD's impact on the extremities can be attributed to several factors, including reduced oxygenation, systemic inflammation, and the side effects of chronic respiratory distress.

These factors can lead to noticeable changes and conditions affecting the extremities, offering important clues for diagnosis. These include some of the skin manifestations we've seen above, which occur on the skin of the upper and lower extremities first.

This is because the extremities are located furthest from the heart, making them the last to receive oxygenated blood. When oxygen levels in the blood decrease, they are the first to exhibit signs of inadequate oxygen supply, such as fatigue and coldness.

Additionally, when there is a shortage in oxygen supply, the body begins to prioritize vital organs, which further reduces the levels of oxygen in the limbs.

Upper and lower extremity symptoms are:

- Clubbing
- Peripheral edema
- Cyanosis of the heart
- Cold extremities (hands and feet feeling cold to the touch)

The extremities may also suffer two additional symptoms, which are caused by the insufficient oxygenation of arms, legs, hands, and feet. These include:

- **Muscle wasting and weakness.** Reduced physical activity levels due to breathing difficulties, coupled with systemic inflammation, can lead to muscle wasting and weakness, particularly noticeable in the extremities.

  This muscle atrophy also contributes to the cycle of decreased mobility and further deconditioning, leading to further endurance and strength decline.

- **Peripheral neuropathy (PN).** PN in COPD primarily occurs due to chronic hypoxemia, where prolonged low levels of oxygen in the blood impair nerve function, and cause nerve damage or death.

  The body's inflammatory response to COPD, along with vascular issues stemming from the disease, can further contribute to the development of PN. Symptoms typically include tingling sensations, numbness, pain, and weakness in the hands and feet, often leading to difficulty with balance and coordination.

  PN is one of the most common comorbidities of COPD, with an incidence of COPD patients of 5 to 100%. Estimations show that two-thirds of patients with COPD show physical signs of PN.

Although, alone, each of these conditions is not indicative of COPD, they prove the systemic nature of this respiratory disease, and its power to negatively affect several body systems, from the lungs to the cardiovascular and nervous systems.

Chest And Lungs

The chest and lungs are the primary sites affected in COPD, where it causes pathological changes that lead to the symptoms commonly associated with this condition, including persistent cough and shortness of breath.

The **manifestations in the chest and lungs result from chronic inflammation, airflow limitation, and the progressive destruction of lung parenchyma** (the breakdown or damage to the tissue in the lungs where gas exchange occurs, compromising respiratory efficiency).

These changes lead to the following symptoms:

- **Barrel chest:** This is a characteristic of advanced stages of COPD and describes a condition in which the anterior-posterior diameter of the chest increases. This change is due to the hyperinflation of the lungs and air trapping that accompany emphysema (a subtype of COPD that involves the destruction of air sacs in the lungs).

  Following these changes, the chest diameter increases in an effort to maintain airflow despite obstructed airways, giving it the characteristic "barrel" shape.

- **Diminished breath sounds:** During auscultation, healthcare providers may note decreased breath sounds in individuals with COPD. This symptom arises because of the reduced air movement through the narrowed or obstructed airways, and the presence of mucus may further dampen the sound.

- **Wheezing:** The presence of high-pitched sounds, especially on exhalation, can indicate significant airflow limitation, a symptom of COPD.

- **Prolonged expiration:** A prolonged expiratory phase during breathing is another hallmark of COPD, often observed during the physical examination. This phenomenon occurs because the narrowed or partly obstructed airways create resistance to airflow, making it difficult for the patient to fully exhale the air from their lungs.

Takeaways

- COPD manifests as airflow limitation from chronic inflammation and tissue destruction in the lungs. Because of its systemic nature, its impact extends to multiple systems, organs, and tissues.
- The GOLD standard categorizes COPD into four stages - mild, moderate, severe, and end-stage - based on symptoms, lung function, and complications.
- Early signs include persistent cough, sputum production, and breathlessness, primarily during physical activity.
- Systemic effects of COPD encompass a decline in physical stamina, weight loss, muscle wasting, increased anxiety, depression, impaired sleep, and cognitive functions due to reduced oxygen levels.
- Skin manifestations of COPD include cyanosis (bluish discoloration), peripheral edema (swelling), and clubbing (bulbous fingers). These symptoms reflect disease severity and chronic hypoxemia.
- Peripheral edema in COPD signals potential cor pulmonale, a serious condition related to right heart failure.
- Symptoms in the upper and lower extremities, including muscle weakness and peripheral neuropathy, indicate poor oxygenation and systemic inflammation.
- The chest and lungs exhibit specific physical signs like barrel chest, diminished breath sounds, wheezing, and prolonged expiration due to advanced COPD.
- This chapter highlights the importance of recognizing the broad and systemic nature of COPD, beyond just respiratory symptoms.
- Early diagnosis and comprehensive management are crucial to mitigate the systemic impacts of COPD and improve quality of life.

Chapter 5 - Airway Obstruction: COPD's Potential Impact On Lung Function And Health

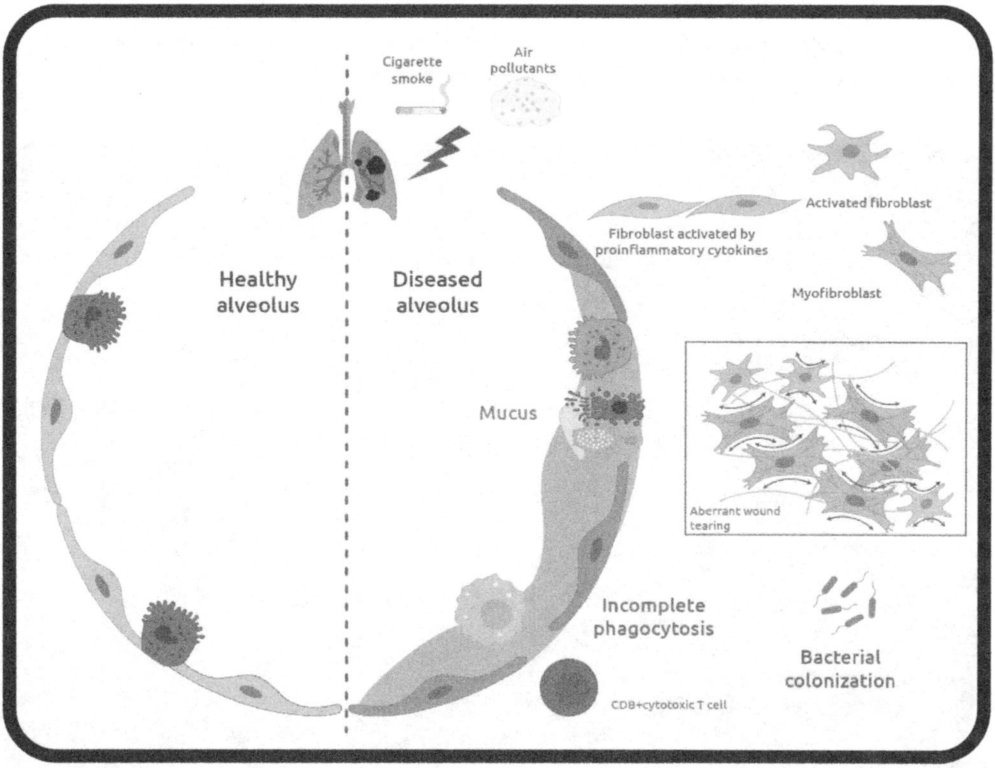

Airway obstruction and inflammatory cells involved in COPD.

Data from: https://www.researchgate.net/figure/Airway-obstruction-and-inflammatory-cells-involved-in-COPD-In-chronic-obstructive_fig2_357605189

Above, I've talked you through the manifestations of COPD on the chest and lungs, and we've covered the manifestations of this disease in the respiratory system, as well as across the body.

However, to better understand the systemic impact of COPD, it is important to **identify the primary villain of the story:** airway obstruction. Far beyond being just a symptom, airway obstruction is the root cause of a whole host of complications of COPD, including emphysema and chronic (long-term) bronchitis.

Obstruction of the airways in COPD is usually caused by ongoing inflammation, which is persistent and capable of causing gradual but significant changes in the lungs. This compromises your ability to breathe and your lungs' capacity for exchanging gas and distributing oxygen to the various organs, cells, and tissues.

Silent killer: A look into the development of inflammation in the lungs.

Initially, the inflammation irritates the lining of the airways. Over time, this irritation leads to a thickening of the walls, reducing the airways' diameter and making it harder for air to flow in and out. But the story doesn't end here.

The inflammation also damages the lung tissue, affecting its elasticity and the functionality of air sacs. When this happens, the lungs' natural architecture is altered, affecting their ability to transfer oxygen to the blood and remove carbon dioxide.

This causes a cascade of events and complications, including:

- The air sacs (alveoli) deteriorate and lose their structure, leading to less surface area for gas exchange.
- The airways become inflamed and filled with mucus, further obstructing airflow.
- The systemic inflammation begins to impact the functioning of the respiratory system as a whole and damage tissues and organs.
- In an effort to fight inflammation, the body can begin to experience increased fatigue and decreased immunity.

It is also important to understand the role of the immune system in the development of COPD. Studies have dubbed the immune system in this scenario both "a victim and an aggressor." This is because the damaging high levels of inflammation are, in fact, caused by the body's immune response.

At the same time, such high levels of inflammation impair the immune system as a whole - so much so, that often, people with COPD are considered immunocompromised. Their immune system is weakened and unable to fight infections, which exposes patients to further risks of disease and infection.

In the sections below, we'll look at the causes and implications of two main types of COPD: **emphysema-predominant and obstruction-predominant COPD.** Here's an overview of the differences before diving deeper into this topic:

- **Emphysema-predominant COPD.** Emphysema-predominant COPD is characterized by damage to the alveoli, the tiny, balloon-like air sacs in the lungs. This form leads to emphysema, or a decrease in respiratory surface area, impairing oxygen exchange.

  Patients with this type of COPD often experience breathlessness and a decreased ability to exercise. The primary culprits include years of exposure to cigarette smoke or other irritants that compromise the architecture of the lungs.

- **Airway obstruction-predominant COPD.** Airway obstruction-predominant COPD, on the other hand, is characterized by chronic bronchitis. In this type of COPD, the bronchial tubes, responsible for carrying air into and out of your lungs, become inflamed and narrowed.

  The hallmarks of this disease include a persistent cough with mucus production and frequent respiratory infections. Although airway obstruction-predominant COPD may have a range of causes and risk factors, it often stems from a chronic inflammatory response to airway irritants.

According to studies, patients with emphysema-predominant COPD have a greater five-year mortality and a worse annual decline in lung function than airway obstruction-predominant COPD.

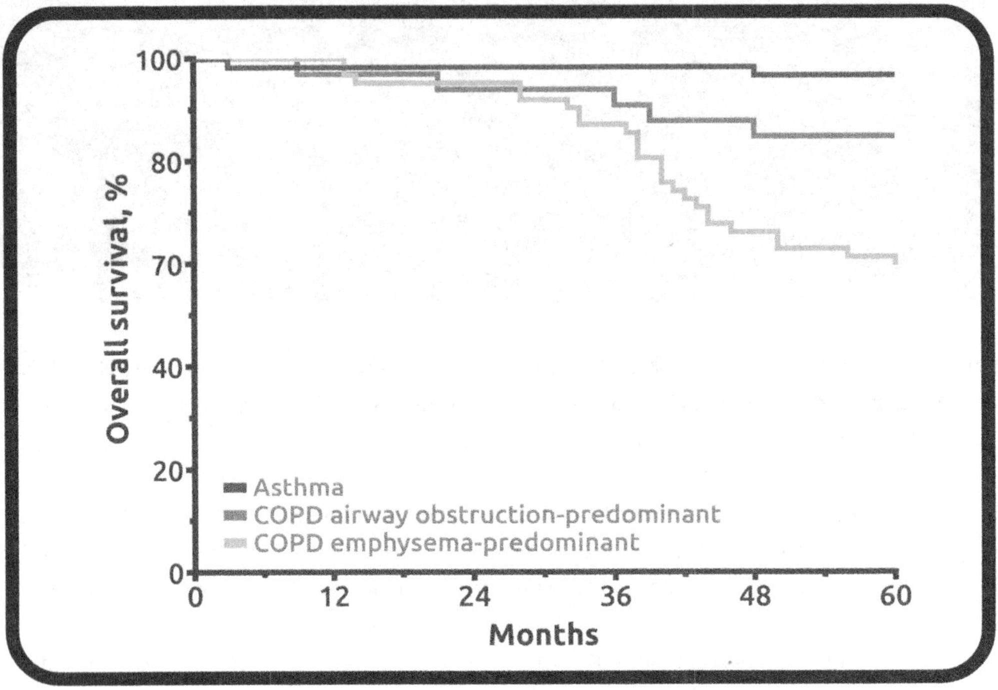

Kaplan–Meier survival curves for matched asthma and COPD cohort for five-year all-cause mortality.

Data from: https://www.ncbi.nlm.nih.gov/pmc/articles/PMC8622286/

However, both conditions require immediate care and intervention to prevent complications down the line. And, of course, understanding which of the two types of COPD you are dealing with is the first step to finding a treatment plan that works for your needs.

Emphysema

Emphysema originates from the Greek word "emphysan," meaning "to inflate." This respiratory condition is characterized by damage to the alveoli (air sacs) in the lungs, leading to breathlessness. It falls under the umbrella of chronic obstructive pulmonary diseases.

These **alveoli play a crucial role in facilitating the processes necessary for gas exchange:** they are where oxygen enters the blood and carbon dioxide exits. When emphysema takes root, these sacs are gradually destroyed, leading to decreased surface area. Decreased surface area means that less oxygen can be taken in and less carbon dioxide disposed of. In turn, this impairs oxygen exchange and inhibits the lungs' ability to oxygenate the blood.

Emphysema is primarily **a result of long-term, persistent inflammation in the lungs.** There can be many causes for this chronic inflammation, including genetic factors. However, in the majority of cases, persistent inflammation can be attributed to lifestyle and environmental factors. These include smoking, inhaling cigarette smoke, and exposure to toxins and irritants.

Over time, this inflammation leads to structural changes within the lung and damage to the walls of the air sacs. The more air sacs are destroyed, the less efficient the gas exchange becomes. At the same time, the lungs begin to become less elastic, making it increasingly difficult for the individual to breathe out fully, leading to air trapping and reduced airflow. These are two of the key symptoms of COPD.

Here are key factors about emphysema to keep in mind:

- **Emphysema is a subtype of COPD, alongside chronic bronchitis.** A person diagnosed with COPD may have both conditions. However, often, the presence and severity of emphysema are used as indicators to determine the impact of the condition on lung function. This indicator can also tell a lot about a patient's prognosis.

- **Globally, the prevalence of emphysema is challenging to pinpoint** due to variances in diagnostic criteria and reporting. However, it is estimated that millions of individuals worldwide are living with this condition.

- **The leading cause of emphysema is smoking.** The CDC estimates that it affects over 15% of current cigarette smokers, nearly 7.6% of former smokers, and nearly 3% of never smokers. Other factors, such as genetic predispositions (e.g., alpha-1 antitrypsin deficiency) and environmental and occupational exposures contribute to the development of emphysema but are not seen as direct causes.

- **The prognosis of emphysema** is linked to the stage at which it is diagnosed and how well the contributing factors, particularly smoking, are managed. Early detection and cessation of smoking can significantly slow the progression, improving quality of life. However, the damage already caused to the lungs is irreversible. This means that treatments will focus on preventing further damage and managing symptoms.

Chronic (Long-Term) Bronchitis

Chronic bronchitis is defined by the persistent inflammation of the bronchial tubes, which serve as the airways that carry air into your lungs. This condition is characterized by distinct symptoms, like a daily cough and mucus (sputum) production for at least three months in a year, for two consecutive years.

The chronic inflammation leads to swelling and increased mucus production. As mucus begins to build up, it obstructs the air flow in and out of the lungs. As the airflow is reduced, the typical symptoms of COPD appear, including chronic cough and difficult breathing.

Key information about chronic bronchitis to keep in mind include:

- **Chronic bronchitis often develops due to prolonged exposure to irritants** that damage the lungs and airways. Cigarette smoke is the most common culprit, but exposure to air pollution, dust, and toxic gasses in the environment or workplace also plays a significant role.

Risk Factor	Association
Cigarette Smoking	Strong
Occupational Exposures:	Moderate
1- Coal miners	
2- Hard-rock miners	
3- Tunnel workers	
4- Concrete manufacturers	
5- Livestock farming	
Exposure to Agricultural Pesticides	Moderate
Use of Domestic Solid Fuels	Moderate
Electronic Cigarettes	Weak
Marijuana Smoking	Weak
Air Pollution	Weak

Risk Factors for Developing CB and COPD

Data from: https://www.ncbi.nlm.nih.gov/pmc/articles/PMC6596437/

- **Estimates suggest that millions of people worldwide** - approximately 10 million people in the United States alone - suffer from chronic bronchitis, with a higher prevalence among smokers, individuals over the age of 45, and those exposed to significant levels of environmental or occupational irritants.

- **The prognosis for chronic bronchitis** relies on several factors, including:

  - The severity at diagnosis
  - The patient's smoking status
  - Exposure to other lung irritants

  Early detection and intervention can significantly alter the disease's trajectory and prevent further damage.

- **Preventive measures and lifestyle modifications,** as we'll see in the upcoming chapters, play a vital role in reducing the risk of further damage. In particular, smoking cessation is paramount for those diagnosed, as continuing to smoke can accelerate the disease's progression and worsen the prognosis.

Chronic bronchitis falls under the umbrella of COPD, alongside emphysema. While the two conditions have their distinct features, they often coexist, and many individuals with COPD have elements of both.

Takeaways

- Airway obstruction is a central aspect of COPD, leading to complications like emphysema and chronic bronchitis.
- Persistent inflammation in the airways causes thickening and narrowing, making it difficult for air to flow, leading to decreased lung function.
- COPD is marked by a downward spiral, where inflammation in the lungs affects tissue elasticity and air sac structure, which, in turn, impairs gas exchange.
- The immune system plays a dual role in COPD as both a victim and aggressor, contributing to inflammation and becoming compromised over time.
- Emphysema-predominant COPD primarily results from damage to the alveoli, reducing the lungs' capacity for oxygen exchange and leading to breathlessness.
- Airway obstruction-predominant COPD is characterized by chronic bronchitis, with symptoms of persistent cough and mucus production due to inflamed airways.
- Emphysema's root cause is long-term inflammation, often from smoking or exposure to air pollutants, which leads to irreversible changes in the lungs' structure.
- The prognosis and management of emphysema and chronic bronchitis depend on early detection, cessation of smoking, and managing other contributing factors.

Chapter 6 - The Essential Role of Prevention In COPD

As I have said above, in COPD, genetic factors play only a small part. This means that **the majority of contributors and causes derive from lifestyle and environment and are, therefore, modifiable.** Given this assumption, it is easy to see how implementing preventive strategies early on can help individuals - whether at risk of COPD or not - take control of their respiratory health and reduce the risk of pulmonary conditions.

In particular, preventive efforts are important both in healthy individuals and in patients who have been diagnosed with COPD. Even though preventive measures may not be able to reverse the damage inflicted to the lungs by inflammation or "cure" the disease, they certainly play a major role in helping patients live with COPD. Here are some of the goals of a preventive plan:

- **Slowing the disease's progression.** COPD is inherently progressive, meaning it can worsen over time. By adopting preventive measures, individuals can manage the speed at which the disease advances, potentially preserving lung function and maintaining independence and healthspan for longer.

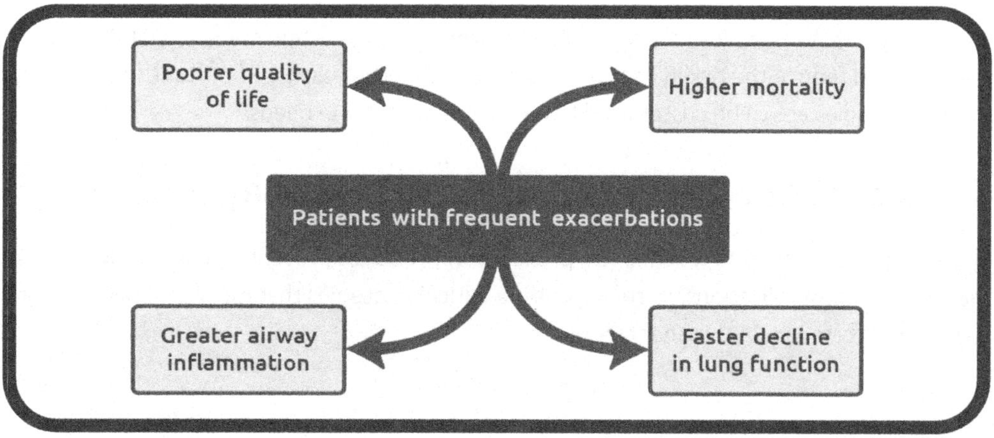

Effect of COPD exacerbations in the group with frequent exacerbation

Data from: https://www.ncbi.nlm.nih.gov/pmc/articles/PMC7134993/figure/fig2/

- **Reducing the frequency and severity of exacerbations.** In the sections above, I've talked about exacerbations. These are acute periods when symptoms become significantly and rapidly worse than their usual day-to-day variation, affecting morbidity and mortality. These exacerbations can be triggered by factors like infections, high stress levels, or even the seasonal flu. Not only do they impair quality of life but also contribute to the overall decline in lung function. Nonetheless, preventing exacerbation is possible with lifestyle and environmental modifications.

- **Mitigating the risk of complications.** From respiratory infections to heart problems, COPD can lead to a host of serious complications. Through proactive prevention, the risk of these complications can be reduced. While this may not "cure" the disease, it can help patients better live with COPD.

- **Enhancing the general well-being and quality of life for individuals with COPD.** Unaddressed, COPD will, over time, affect your ability to perform daily activities, work, or live independently, which can lead to a fast decline in physical health as well as mental health conditions, like social isolation, depression, and anxiety. Studies have confirmed that people with COPD have a higher risk of dementia and cognitive impairment. That's where preventive measures can help. By preventing complications and exacerbations of the disease, preventive efforts can improve a person's health span and quality of life, reducing the risk of disability, surgery, and hospitalization.

Below, we'll look in detail at the preventive strategies that can help manage COPD in patients and reduce the risk in healthy individuals. Nonetheless, it is important to notice that these strategies are to be customized to each patient's unique needs:

Preventive Strategies In COPD Management

Managing COPD effectively requires a proactive approach to prevent exacerbations, or flare-ups, and complications. Here, we outline critical strategies that form the backbone of preemptive care in COPD management:

- **Smoking cessation.** If you smoke, the single most effective strategy for preventing COPD progression and exacerbations is to quit smoking or reduce your intake. You may also consider modifying your environment so that you are not regularly exposed to secondhand smoke, which can be just as damaging. As you know by now, smoking irritates and inflames the lungs, accelerating lung damage, leading to what's known as "smoker's cough," and making flare-ups more likely. Quitting smoking can halt damage and prevent further deterioration of lung function.

- **Avoiding air pollutants.** Environmental and occupational pollutants can exacerbate COPD symptoms. If you live or work in an environment where you may be regularly exposed to dust, chemical fumes, and air pollution, you may be advised to modify your lifestyle or use personal protective equipment (PPE). In high-pollution areas or during poor air quality days, staying indoors or wearing protective masks can help mitigate risks. Occupational COPD is underdiagnosed: it is estimated that around 70% of persistent airflow obstruction cases are not diagnosed due to limited use of diagnostic instruments and under-recognition of at-risk demographics (e.g.: young people, never smokers, and workers - those who are theoretically less likely to develop COPD). Pollutants to be avoided include:

  - Asbestos
  - Volatile organic compounds (VOCs)
  - Dust
  - Chemical fumes and ash
  - Aerosol paint
  - Pesticide
  - Cleaning chemicals
  - Fossil fuels used for cooking
  - Exhaust and diesel fumes
  - Sensitizers

- **Vaccination.** Influenza and pneumococcal vaccines greatly reduce the risk of respiratory infections, which are known triggers for COPD exacerbations. If you are at risk of COPD or you are looking to manage the damage caused to lungs by exacerbations, annual flu shots and timely pneumococcal vaccinations as recommended can boost your defenses against these common but potentially severe infections.

- **Regular exercise.** Tailored exercise programs help strengthen respiratory muscles, improving endurance and lung capacity, and reducing symptoms. Even a moderate activity level, adjusted to the patient's abilities, can enhance lung efficiency and reduce the frequency of exacerbations.

- **Adherence to your treatment plan.** Long-term and rescue medications (medications taken to alleviate symptoms during flare-ups) represent a critical part of COPD management. They are used to reduce inflammation and open airways. Because of this, the correct use of inhalers and adherence to prescribed treatment regimens can help you keep symptoms under control and prevent exacerbations.

Besides these preventive strategies, you should also speak to your doctor to learn to recognize the early signs of exacerbations. You and your doctors may also strategize an action plan that will allow you to act fast when the first symptoms appear, thus reducing the risk for further, much more threatening complications.

Some actions your healthcare providers may recommend you take upon the early signs of an exacerbation include:

- Increase use of inhalers as prescribed.
- Initiate prescribed oral steroids or antibiotics.
- Use supplemental oxygen if prescribed.
- Seek immediate medical attention if symptoms worsen.
- Follow an action plan developed with a healthcare provider.
- Stay hydrated and avoid known triggers (e.g.: stress or extreme weather events).

Remember, early intervention can prevent a mild exacerbation from becoming severe.

Takeaways

- Preventive strategies in COPD focus on slowing disease progression, reducing exacerbation frequency, minimizing complications, and enhancing quality of life.
- Smoking cessation is the most effective way to halt COPD progression and prevent exacerbations.
- Avoiding air pollutants, including chemicals, dust, and fumes, is crucial in managing COPD symptoms and preventing flare-ups.
- Regular vaccinations, such as the flu and pneumococcal vaccines, can significantly reduce the risk of respiratory infections that trigger COPD exacerbations.
- Tailored exercise programs strengthen respiratory muscles, improving lung efficiency and reducing symptom frequency.
- Adhering to prescribed treatment plans and properly using inhalers can help in controlling COPD symptoms and preventing exacerbations.
- Early recognition and management of exacerbation signs can prevent severe complications and the need for hospitalization. It is also important to have an action plan in place to execute when the first signs of exacerbation occur.

Chapter 7 - Diagnosing COPD

A 2019 study published in the International Journal of Chronic Obstructive Pulmonary Disease clearly states:

> *"Late COPD diagnosis is associated with higher exacerbation rate and increased comorbidities and costs compared with early diagnosis."*

However, as I shared with you early on in this book, people don't notice the symptoms until they get worse. As a consequence, most patients seek an adequate diagnosis only when they are already in the second or even third stage of the disease.

Nonetheless, if you suspect that you are at risk of COPD because of genetics, due to your personal and professional circumstances, or because you are a smoker, you can tackle this disease early on by getting the necessary screening tests. In particular, your doctor may help you better understand your risk of this disease and evaluate your symptoms by carrying out an **evaluation of your medical history and a comprehensive physical examination.**

These initial steps are crucial because they offer the first clues about the presence of COPD and help guide the direction of subsequent, more specialized diagnostic tests. Given the fact that neither of these evaluations are uncomfortable or painful, there's no reason why patients at risk should miss out on annual screening tests. Here's what to expect:

- **Medical history review.** During a medical history review, you'll have a detailed conversation with your doctor, during which they will inquire about:
  - Your symptoms, such as chronic cough, shortness of breath, and wheezing
  - Smoking history, given its significant role in COPD development
  - Exposure to lung irritants like pollution, dust, and chemicals
  - Family history of respiratory diseases, which can predispose individuals to COPD

- **Physical examination:** Here, the doctor will carry out a physical examination to determine the presence of signs indicative of COPD. These tests include:
    - Observing your general appearance
    - Looking for signs of respiratory distress
    - Listening to the lungs with a stethoscope for telltale sounds like wheezing, crackles, or reduced breath noises
    - Checking for signs of cyanosis, which could indicate low oxygen levels

If your doctor suspects that you have COPD or another respiratory condition, they may recommend that you undergo more specific tests. These tests are needed to confirm the diagnosis and determine the severity of your condition by examining indicators (e.g.: how extensive the emphysema is).

Laboratory Tests

The symptoms of COPD that are outwardly visible are often non-specific. Think of wheezing, coughing, or shortness of breath: they can indicate an infection or be easily confused with other conditions, such as asthma or heart failure.

That is why, to accurately diagnose COPD and distinguish it from these other conditions, your doctor may recommend one or more laboratory tests to gain insights into your lung health and function.

These tests include:

- **Spirometry.** Initially introduced in 1846, spirometry is still today the cornerstone of COPD diagnosis. This test employs a spirometer and aims to measure the quantity and speed of air a patient can exhale. Comparing this indicator against normal values can help identify airflow obstruction, a symptom of COPD. Physicians rely on this test to assess the severity of the condition and to monitor its progression or response to treatment.

- **Alpha-1 antitrypsin deficiency testing.** Alpha-1 antitrypsin deficiency is a genetic condition that can lead to COPD, even in patients who have never smoked, by weakening the lungs and respiratory system. Testing for this deficiency is essential, especially if COPD develops at a younger age or in non-smokers, as it can influence treatment strategies. Given the genetic nature of this condition, knowing your risk is also important to inform family members about their likelihood of developing COPD.

- **Chest X-ray.** Although this test isn't specifically recommended to diagnose COPD, a chest X-ray can reveal signs of lung hyperinflation or rule out other lung conditions such as pneumonia or lung cancer. It's a useful tool in the diagnostic process, helping clinicians to eliminate other potential causes of the patient's symptoms and confirm their assumptions.

- **Oximetry.** This non-invasive test measures the oxygen saturation levels in the blood. Oximetry test results are used as indicators of how well oxygen is being transported to the extremities farthest from the heart. Low oxygen levels can suggest the presence of COPD or another lung disease that may be impairing oxygen circulation, which may warrant further investigation.

- **CT scan.** Computed tomography (CT) scans provide detailed images of the lungs. They are extremely helpful because they can show emphysema, one of the components of COPD, even before symptoms become obvious. CT scans are particularly useful in planning treatment, identifying complications, or assessing the severity of the disease or how well it responds to treatment.

- **Arterial blood gas analysis.** This test measures the oxygen and carbon dioxide levels in the arterial blood, giving insight into how well the lungs are capable of exchanging gas. In COPD patients, this indicator can describe the extent to which COPD affects breathing efficiency. In turn, it is crucial for gauging the disease's severity and guiding oxygen therapy if necessary.

Although you may not need to undergo all of these tests, your doctor may recommend one or more of these to accurately determine what's affecting your respiratory system, as well as the extent and severity of the disease.

Takeaways

- Recognizing early symptoms of COPD is crucial, but these often go unnoticed until later stages of the disease. Because of this, the importance of regular screening for those at risk cannot be overstated.
- Initial diagnosis begins with a comprehensive review of medical history and a physical examination, focusing on symptoms, smoking history, and exposure to lung irritants.
- Specialized tests like spirometry, alpha-1 antitrypsin deficiency testing, chest X-ray, oximetry, CT scans, and arterial blood gas analysis are essential for confirming COPD diagnosis and understanding its severity.
- Spirometry remains the foundational test for diagnosing COPD, measuring airflow obstruction and function.
- Testing for alpha-1 antitrypsin deficiency is vital for patients with COPD symptoms, especially if they are non-smokers or diagnosed at a young age.
- Imaging tests and blood gas analysis play significant roles in eliminating other conditions, assessing the extent of lung damage, and guiding treatment plans.

Chapter 8 - Conventional Treatment Options

COPD treatment and management plans have evolved significantly since the disease first became a recognized medical condition. As technology and healthcare have advanced in leaps and bounds since the late 1840s, today's patients can access an array of treatment options, which reflect these advances in pulmonary medicine.

Modern treatment options for COPD range from medications like bronchodilators and steroids to interventions such as pulmonary rehabilitation and various surgical procedures including bullectomy, lung volume reduction surgery, and lung transplantation.

However, it is crucial to acknowledge that these treatments come with their own set of downsides and risks. Given that COPD is a chronic and progressive disease without a cure, the primary aim of these treatments is to manage and alleviate symptoms and improve quality of life.

Although they may help with slowing disease progression, they are inefficient in resolving it. Consequently, patients often find themselves navigating the potential risk of medication side effects or the inherent risks associated with surgical interventions.

This complex treatment landscape tell us that:

A) Treatment plans should be entirely tailored to the patient's needs.
B) Medications and surgery may not be long-term sustainable ways to address COPD.
C) It is critical to look beyond conventional treatments to seek interventions that are less risky, safer, and more sustainable in the long term.

Medications

The treatment of COPD relies heavily on medications to alleviate symptoms, improve quality of life, and decrease the frequency of flare-ups. These medications fall into several categories, each targeting different aspects of the disease. Here are some of the interventions more commonly recommended by healthcare providers:

- **Bronchodilators.** These are often considered the foundation of any COPD treatment plan. They are medications containing substances like beta2-agonists or anticholinergics, which can be inhaled to relax and widen the airways' muscles, helping to keep them open for easier breathing. They come in two main types:

  - Short-acting bronchodilators (e.g., albuterol) provide quick relief from acute symptoms. They are rescue medications.
  - Long-acting bronchodilators (e.g., tiotropium, salmeterol) are used daily to maintain the airways open in time. They are maintenance medications.

  Research indicates that inhaled therapy can help with long-term prevention of COPD by reducing exacerbation frequency and intensity.

- **Corticosteroids.** Inhaled corticosteroids (like fluticasone and budesonide) help reduce inflammation in the airways. Additionally, by inhibiting the immune system's inflammatory pathways, they reduce swelling and mucus production in the airways, making breathing easier and helping to prevent future flare-ups. They are often prescribed along with long-acting bronchodilators for more severe forms of COPD.

- **Phosphodiesterase-4 inhibitors.** Phosphodiesterase-4 inhibitors like roflumilast, often referred to by the brand names Daxas or Daliresp, is a medication that targets inflammation in a different way compared to corticosteroids, by inhibiting an enzyme called phosphodiesterase-4 (PDE-4). This action reduces inflammation and relaxes the airways, improving airflow. Research shows that roflumilast may lead to fewer flare-ups, improved lung function, and better quality of life by directly targeting the inflammation that exacerbates the condition.

- **Antibiotics and antivirals:** These medications can help combat flare-ups, and they are usually used as "rescue" drugs. They may be prescribed during acute exacerbations when infection is present. Since infections can significantly worsen COPD symptoms and lead to hospitalization, antivirals and antibiotics may help the body combat the "invader" and overcome the flare-up quickly, thus preventing complications.

- **Vaccinations.** Vaccinations aren't a treatment for COPD, but flu and pneumonia vaccines are crucial in preventing infections that can exacerbate the condition. The flu vaccine, recommended annually, protects you against the seasonal influenza virus that can cause acute bronchitis and pneumonia, potentially leading to severe COPD flare-ups. The pneumonia vaccine protects against pneumococcal infections, a common cause of pneumonia, which can become dangerous when contracted by a COPD patient with a weakened immune system. Vaccinations also play an important role in safeguarding COPD patients against potentially fatal complications of COVID-19: according to a 2023 study, the prevalence of death in people with both COVID-19 and COPD was 40%.

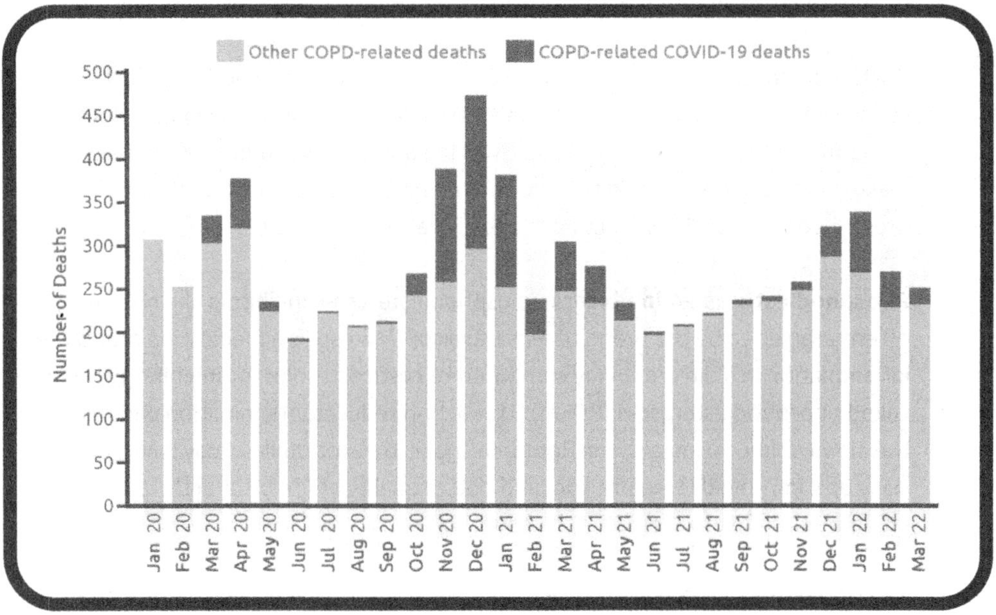

Monthly Number Of Copd-Related Deaths, With And Without Covid-19 As The Underlying Cause.

Data from: https://www.ncbi.nlm.nih.gov/pmc/articles/PMC10459975/

Although these medications - when used alone or in combination - may help patients manage their disease and improve their quality of life, they are not free of side effects. And, since COPD is a progressive, chronic disease, it is important to evaluate the long-term effects on health of taking medications daily.

After all, corticosteroids, antibiotics, or phosphodiesterase-4 inhibitors, when taken regularly, can lead to side effects like weight loss, diarrhea, nausea, and headache, as well as reliance, tolerance, and addiction.

Additionally, studies have started to look into possible alternatives to - or interventions that can help reduce the need for - long-acting bronchodilators and anti-inflammatory drugs. Recent research highlights that there may be easier ways to achieve similar exacerbation prevention using non-pharmacological tools (compared to pharmacological tools).

Lung Therapies

Besides medications, lung therapies are commonly prescribed in the management of moderate and advanced stages of COPD. They play a pivotal role in helping COPD patients improve lung function without additional medications. These therapies include:

- **Pulmonary rehabilitation.** A comprehensive program combining education on lung health, supervised exercise training, coping strategies, nutrition advice, and counseling tailored to enhance the physical and emotional condition of COPD patients. By learning more about their condition and prevention strategies, patients can become more accountable for their pulmonary health, which has been seen to yield positive results. According to studies, pulmonary rehabilitation improves exercise tolerance, reduces breathlessness, increases the distance walked in six minutes, and improves mobility and ability to exercise.

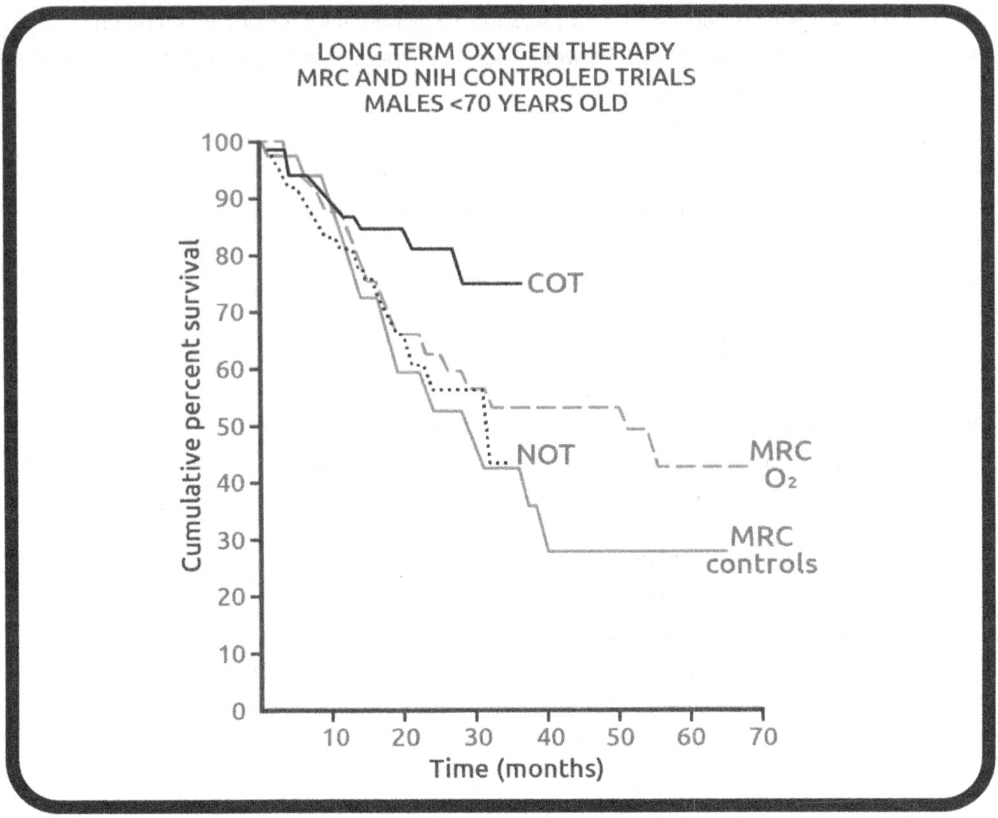

Data from: https://www.ncbi.nlm.nih.gov/pmc/articles/PMC2897694/

- **Oxygen therapy.** Used for individuals with severe COPD and low levels of oxygen in their blood, this therapy can help with breathlessness and improve quality of life. It works by boosting the amount of oxygen in your bloodstream, aiding in easier breathing for those with certain medical conditions, including COPD and asthma. By delivering oxygen through a mask or nasal prongs, it helps ensure your organs function properly and can reduce symptoms and improve quality of life. Although it may not completely resolve breathlessness, it has been seen to improve survival in patients with severe COPD for three years. It may be prescribed for use all the time or only during activities or sleep.

- **Ventilation support.** In advanced cases of COPD, noninvasive positive pressure ventilation (NIPPV) can help reduce the efforts needed for breathing. It works by delivering air to the lungs under pressure through a mask. This method enhances oxygen exchange and supports the respiratory muscles, decreasing their workload, which can significantly benefit those with conditions like COPD by improving ventilation and reducing effort during breathing.

These therapies may be used alone or in combinations in the management of COPD, as prescribed by your healthcare provider and based on your unique needs.

Surgery

In managing COPD, surgery represents a critical option - or a last resort - recommended when other treatments fail to control severe symptoms or complications. The surgical procedures available in the treatment of COPD are many and diverse.

These surgical interventions are considered based on a detailed assessment of the patient to ensure the benefits substantially outweigh the risks. Nonetheless, as we'll cover in the next chapter, COPD management involves risks such as infection, prolonged recovery times, and in some cases, rejection of transplanted tissue.

Additionally, although COPD patients may benefit from surgical interventions, the success rates of these operations should be carefully considered. For example, according to estimations, the survival rate five years after lung volume reduction surgery averages between 63% and 78%.

Below, we'll look at the most commonly prescribed surgical interventions for advanced or end-stage COPD.

Bullectomy

Bullectomy involves the surgical removal of bullae, which are large air pockets within the lungs that obstruct breathing. The removal of these air spaces enables the rest of the lung to expand more effectively, improves oxygen exchange, and lowers the risk of lung infections.

As a result, patients experience notable improvements in respiratory function and overall well-being. The survival rate after this surgery is 100% after five years and 60% after 10 years, making it a relatively safe option for those eligible.

Lung Volume Reduction Surgery

In lung volume reduction surgery, damaged portions of lung tissue are carefully removed.

This procedure aims to enhance lung performance by allowing the remaining, healthier parts of the lung to function more efficiently. It specifically benefits patients suffering from emphysema. This procedure is performed under general anesthesia, either through traditional open surgery or less invasively using video-assisted thoracoscopic surgery (VATS). When carried out correctly, reducing lung size, this surgery aims to improve breathing mechanics, oxygen exchange, and overall respiratory function, thus enhancing their quality of life.

Lung Transplant

For individuals with end-stage COPD, a lung transplant could be an option to consider. This surgery involves replacing one or both diseased lungs with healthy ones from a donor.

A lung transplant can dramatically improve lung function, increase life expectancy, and enhance the quality of life for recipients. However, it requires a lifelong commitment to immunosuppressive medications to prevent organ rejection and entails rigorous, continuous health monitoring. What's more, aside from the complications we'll see in the next chapter, it is worth keeping in mind that people wait an average of two years for a single lung transplant and up to three years for two lungs.

Takeaways

- COPD treatments have evolved, focusing on symptom management and quality of life improvement. However, surgical interventions and pharmacological interventions are not without risks.
- Medications, including bronchodilators and corticosteroids, play a key role in managing COPD but come with potential side effects and long-term health implications.
- Phosphodiesterase-4 inhibitors and vaccines offer targeted treatment and preventive measures against exacerbations and infections but require careful long-term usage consideration.
- Pulmonary rehabilitation, oxygen therapy, and ventilation support offer non-pharmacological ways to improve lung function and reduce symptoms in COPD patients.
- Surgical options like bullectomy, lung volume reduction surgery, and lung transplantation are considered for severe or end-stage COPD when other treatments fail.
- Bullectomy can significantly improve respiratory function by removing obstructive air pockets in the lungs, with a high survival rate post-surgery.
- Lung volume reduction surgery aims to enhance lung efficiency by removing damaged tissue, with potential to improve overall respiratory function and life quality.
- Lung transplantation offers a chance for dramatically improved lung function and quality of life for end-stage COPD patients, though it involves a significant commitment to post-operative care and monitoring.

Chapter 9 - Surgery Risks For COPD Patients

For patients with severe or end-stage COPD, surgery may seem like the only way out. However, surgery should only be seen as the last resort, in case other less invasive treatments have not worked well in helping you manage symptoms.

In fact, despite the advances in medical technologies that have taken place in the past years, surgery still carries significant risks. So, whether it be a bullectomy, lung volume reduction surgery (LVRS), or a lung transplant, understanding the inherent risks and associated factors is critical.

Surgical interventions in COPD patients carry general risks similar to those in the broader population, such as infection, bleeding, and adverse reactions to anesthesia. However, due to the compromised lung and immune system function inherent to COPD, these patients may face an elevated risk of postoperative complications.

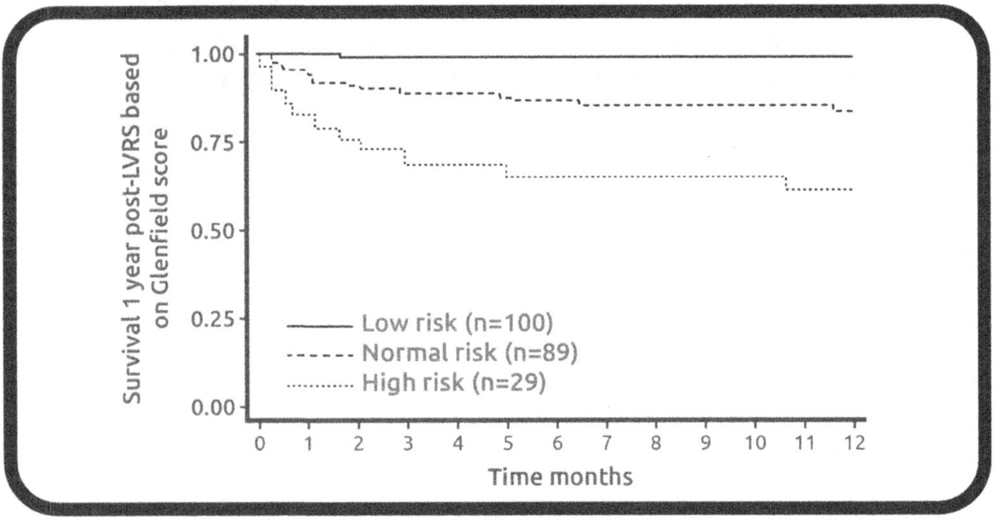

Kaplan–Meier survival of patients up to 1 year post lung volume reduction surgery (LVRS). Survival is shown based on the Glenfield BFG group. Low risk, score 0–1; moderate risk, score 2–3; high risk, score 4–5.

Data from: https://erj.ersjournals.com/content/49/6/1601766

For instance, research indicates that patients undergoing LVRS may experience an improvement in lung function and exercise capacity, but the procedure has a mortality rate of about 5-10% depending on the patients' condition pre-surgery and the experience of the surgeon performing the operation.

Similarly, lung transplants, while potentially life-saving, come with a risk of organ rejection, with about half of the transplants surviving past five years post-surgery. This is because of a condition called chronic lung allograft dysfunction (CLAD), which develops in about 50% of recipients five years after lung transplantation.

This complication, as well as the rising rates of solid organ cancer, is one of the major barriers to long-term survival.

It is also important to note that people with COPD face risks even when undergoing surgeries that aren't aimed at resolving this condition. For example, just requiring general anesthesia can lead to fatal complications like respiratory failure in people with COPD.

Additionally, studies have seen that, in those undergoing non-small cell lung cancer (NSCLC) surgery, having a diagnosis of COPD is a predictor for pulmonary complications.

Beyond the physical risks, the mental impact of awaiting and undergoing surgery for COPD cannot be overestimated. The anticipation of surgery can cause the development of extreme anxiety and fear, not only regarding the outcome but also about the potential for a lengthy and challenging recovery period.

Post-surgery, patients may face months of rehabilitation, during which the fear of possible complications or the surgery failing to produce the right results can feel overwhelming.

It is also important to consider the financial implications of COPD, surgery, and its aftermath. Estimates by the CDC show that people with COPD miss an average of 15 workdays a year, against the 4.5 missed by healthy individuals.

The missed wages are to be summed up to the costs of COPD-specific care and prescription drugs, which amount to over $4300 a year (around a quarter of the non-specific healthcare-related expenses affected by COPD patients, which is $19,449).

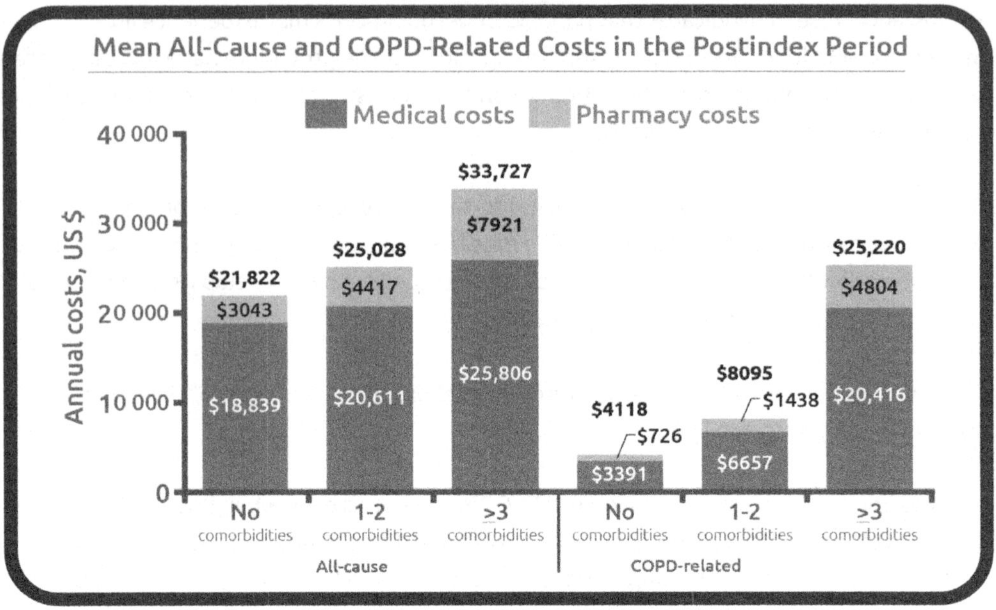

Total All-Cause and COPD-Related Costs by Comorbidity Burden in Patients with Medicare fee-for-service health insurance.

Data from: https://www.ahdbonline.com/articles/3223-the-quality-of-care-and-economic-burden-of-copd-in-the-united-states-considerations-for-managing-patients-and-improving-outcomes

The cost of the surgery itself, coupled with potential income loss from missed workdays during recovery and rehabilitation, can constitute a significant financial burden for many patients and their families.

In summary, while surgical options for COPD can provide crucial benefits for some patients, the decision to proceed requires a comprehensive evaluation of the physical and mental risks, as well as the potential impact on the patient's quality of life and financial well-being.

Careful consideration and discussions with a healthcare provider can help patients navigate these complex decisions and explore alternative treatment options, like stem cells for COPD. Let's look at these alternatives below.

Takeaways

- Surgical options for COPD, including bullectomy and lung transplants, come with substantial risks such as infection and adverse effects from anesthesia. Individuals with COPD also have an increased risk of postoperative complications due to their compromised immune systems.
- The mortality rate for lung volume reduction surgery is between 5-10%, and lung transplant recipients only have a 50% chance of survival past five years, due to complications like organ rejection.
- The anticipation and recovery from surgery can severely impact a patient's mental health and financial stability, due to long recovery periods and the associated costs of surgery and lost income.
- A thorough evaluation of the risks and impacts on quality of life is essential before proceeding with surgery, making it important to consider alternative treatments such as stem cell therapy.

Chapter 10 - Regenerative Alternative: Stem Cell Treatment For COPD

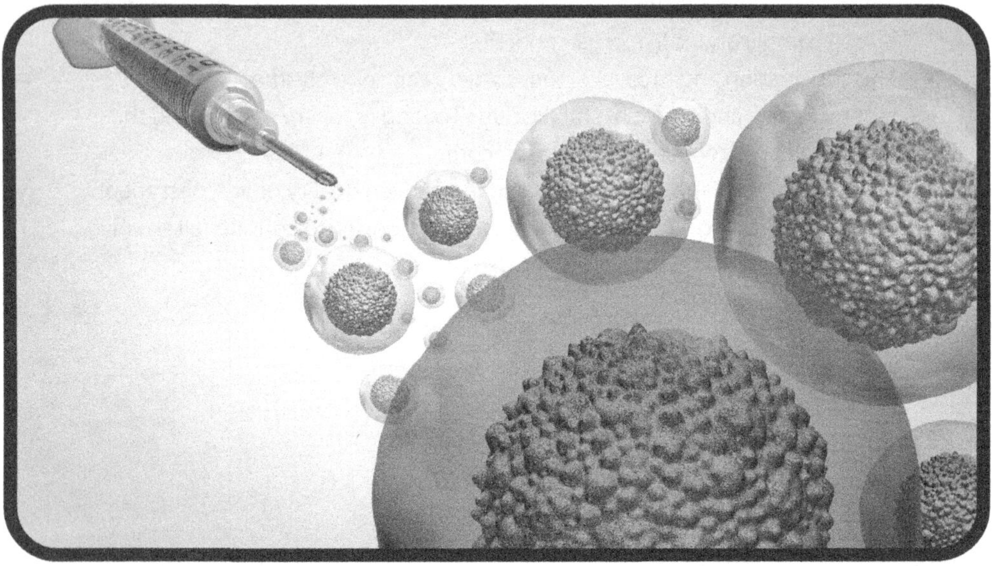

Years ago, in my first biologics lab endeavor, in which we produced birth tissue biologic products that were allowed to be called "stem cells" back then, I noticed a number of physicians and providers asking about the use of our products in IV infusions for treatment of COPD and related symptoms of COPD.

One of the doctors who used our product claimed that he had performed his own IV infusion on himself and that it had produced a noticeably better breathing and respiration effect. He then offered an IV infusion to several of his patients who reported similar outcomes. I was surprised to hear such a general improvement in breathing from so many people.

A couple of years later I learned about an office that was also a client office, offering treatment for COPD using our products. They had simply embraced the success of lung health and breathing and had started offering a treatment for COPD openly.

I was a bit concerned about that idea of openly announcing a treatment option for this condition as I had only ever seen anecdotal evidence of this treatment, but I soon found that multiple offices were actively offering treatment for COPD and seeing great results with dozens of patients.

It soon became apparent that regenerative medicine therapy options may be the only actual viable treatment option for COPD and possibly for other lung conditions like asthma and pulmonary fibrosis.

As of this writing, there are numerous research articles published on the successful progress on using actual genuine mesenchymal stem cells, like the kind I promote that come from your own adipose that are cultured and grown in the lab, for COPD treatment with great results and outcomes.

I am very happy to see the evidence presented in the research on this subject. There is a tremendous potential to treat lung conditions using actual stem cells.

To remind everyone again, the field is very new and though there are great articles coming out showing the use of stem cells in this treatment, it is by no means a refined procedure.

HOWEVER, if you are using your own mesenchymal stem cells collected from your own adipose fat tissue, cultured and expanded and grown into concentrated pure stem cell vials, then the potential for a real therapeutic treatment is definitely possible.

Just to recap what I believe is the best way to do this currently, you will have a small adipose collection procedure performed. This is a small liposuction process and is usually very quick and simple because not very much fat material is needed. It's a 5-10 min process in the office of any skilled and trained plastic surgeon or any medical provider who's been trained in the procedure. Then that sample is shipped to the lab where the stem cells are isolated from everything else.

The process for this is pretty standard procedure for a biotech lab; I've done this sort of thing dozens of times in my biotech career. Next, the cells are introduced to growth plates and growth media fluid and incubated. The growth cycle will continue for weeks.

What you end up with is a culture dish filled with replicated copies of your own mesenchymal stem cells! How amazing is this! You can then reapply those cells to your own body at any time.

This is how I promote the idea of having stem cells for life!!! One collection procedure and you now have stock and inventory of your own pure stem cells for the rest of your life! It's the most amazing development in the stem cell world! Just think about it. If you're 35 years old now and you grow and bank your own cells right now, then you'll have your own 35 year old cells for the rest of your life.

So when you're 75 years old and you want stem cell injections in your knees, you can now use your own cells to do that! You can get regular ongoing stem cell IV infusions and regenerate your whole body. I know people who do this on a quarterly basis and they absolutely swear by it, claiming that they feel and act younger and rejuvenated for months with each infusion.

In fact, they may actually be reducing their biologic age in this process. Possibly creating a situation where they could live well beyond the normal current lifespan.

10 Million PURE Stem Cells vs 10 Million Cells in a Marketing Claim

OK, so anyone who's been pitched stem cells by their doctor or chiropractor has heard the claim of X millions of cells per vial or per injection.

If the doctor is pulling a vial out of the freezer that isn't your own stem cells that you already banked, then what they are pulling out is not stem cells, it's a donated birth tissue slurry injection.

I know this is exactly what it is because I've owned two companies that have made these products. So, what they are calling stem cells is not really stem cells. It's just a bunch of cells.

The claim that you are getting a vial of 10 million cells means you're getting a vial that might have 10 million of something, but not 10 million stem cells. The doctors are woefully misled and miseducated on this fact.

The vial they can buy is not a refined vial of stem cells, it's a refined vial of regular tissue cells that comprise a range of cells, most of which may not even be living and viable: stromal cells, epithelial cells, and connective tissue cells, and maybe a few stem cells. If you're lucky you might have about 2% stem cells in that vial. Maybe.

And if those cells are viable, then maybe those cells will do some good for you. Maybe. BUT that is not a vial of 10 million stem cells, as I have pointed out many times in many books already.

NOW, you have your own refined and grown stem cells and that vial of 10 million cells is true and genuine stem cells! You are absolutely getting a vial of 10 million stem cells because you own them already and you know what it is. It's your own cells.

Think about this: if you get a vial of "not really stem cells" from your doctor and they actually work decently well, think about how much better your own cells will be when you have a vial of 10 million actual stem cells!

Assuming you actually did get 2% viable stem cells in that previous vial, your own pure vial is 100% stem cells, so you are getting a 50 fold increase in actual stem cells from that other injection versus this injection of your own cells!

The Effect Of Stem Cells In Lung Capillary Beds and Their Role in Therapeutic Outcomes

OK, so how does this treatment actually work to help COPD? Well, as I've researched and read in the literature, the cells are passing through the capillary beds of the lungs where a great number of the cells are going to be captured and absorbed into the tissue of the lungs at that point.

OK, so how does this treatment actually work to help COPD? Well, as I've researched and read in the literature, the cells are passing through the capillary beds of the lungs where a great number of the cells are going to be captured and absorbed into the tissue of the lungs at that point.

In fact, this is actually a problem for offering therapy in many scenarios where you need the cells to end up in a distal arterial supply point like down to the lower extremities or other areas, because a great deal of your cell content is captured in the lungs, and of course as you now know, in previous products that aren't your own cells, that vial of product may be lucky to have 2% stem cells, so losing any portion to the capillary beds of the lungs greatly reduced the delivered product load to the extremities.

HOWEVER, this is exactly why this treatment may work so well for COPD and other lung conditions. It's rejuvenating all the lung tissue in great detail because so much cell material and stimulation is occurring in the lungs.

With that said, one intriguing aspect of stem cell therapy now being researched is the observation that infused stem cells often localize in the capillary beds of the lungs. This localization is thought to play a crucial role in the therapeutic effects observed in lung diseases.

The papers I have cited in this section explore the mechanisms by which stem cells are captured in the lung capillary beds and how this phenomenon contributes to the positive outcomes seen in lung function following stem cell infusions.

Mechanisms of Stem Cell Capture in Lung Capillaries: A few more details

When stem cells are infused intravenously, they travel through the bloodstream and are naturally filtered by the capillary beds of the lungs. This phenomenon, known as "pulmonary first-pass effect," occurs because the lungs are the first major organ the cells encounter after entering the venous circulation.

The capillary network in the lungs is extensive and has a high surface area, providing a large interface for cells to interact with the endothelium.

Cellular Adhesion and Mechanotransduction: How stem cells enact benefit

Stem cells, particularly mesenchymal stem cells (MSCs), express a variety of adhesion molecules that interact with the endothelial cells of the lung capillaries. These interactions involve integrins, selectins, and chemokine receptors, facilitating the retention of MSCs in the lung tissue.

Additionally, the mechanical properties of the lung microenvironment, such as shear stress and the structural characteristics of the capillary network, contribute to the physical trapping and retention of stem cells.

- **Stem Cell Size and Deformability:** The relatively large size of MSCs compared to red blood cells causes them to become lodged in the narrow capillaries of the lungs. Their size and deformability, shape altering capacity, mean they can be trapped more easily than smaller or more flexible cells, ensuring they remain in the lung tissue for a prolonged period.

Therapeutic Effects Mediated by Lung Capillary Capture: Multiple reasons and ways that stem cells may create benefit to lung tissues

As I write about these aspects of therapeutic effect, I'm thinking of multiple additional studies that can be conducted in the field. I truly hope to be a part of several of these in the future.

The capture of stem cells in the lung capillaries is not merely a passive process but has significant therapeutic implications. The localization of stem cells in the lung microenvironment facilitates several key mechanisms that contribute to their therapeutic effects.

- **Paracrine Signaling:** One of the primary ways that mesenchymal stem cells exert their therapeutic effects is through the secretion of a wide range of bioactive molecules, including growth factors, cytokines, and extracellular vesicles, also known as exosomes.

  These paracrine signals can modulate the local immune response, reduce inflammation, and promote tissue repair. The close proximity of MSCs to damaged lung tissue ensures that these signals are delivered directly where they are most needed.

- **Immune Modulation:** MSCs have potent immunomodulatory properties. They can alter the behavior of various immune cells, including T cells, B cells, macrophages, and dendritic cells, leading to a reduction in chronic inflammation and autoimmunity. This immunomodulation is particularly beneficial in COPD, where chronic inflammation plays a key role in disease progression.

- **Angiogenesis and Tissue Regeneration:** MSCs secrete factors that promote angiogenesis, the formation of new blood vessels, which is crucial for repairing damaged lung tissue and restoring normal function. Additionally, MSCs can differentiate into various cell types, including epithelial cells and fibroblasts, contributing directly to tissue regeneration.

Evidence from Scientific Research: A couple of additional studies

Several studies have demonstrated the importance of lung capillary capture in the therapeutic effects of stem cell infusions. For example, a study by Fischer et al. (2009) showed that intravenously infused MSCs in a mouse model of lung injury were predominantly retained in the lung capillaries, where they mediated significant reductions in inflammation and promoted tissue repair.

Another study by Lee et al. (2011) highlighted that MSCs delivered intravenously in a rat model of COPD localized primarily in the lungs and led to improved lung function and reduced emphysema.

Moreover, a clinical trial by Weiss et al. (2013) demonstrated that autologous MSC infusion in COPD patients resulted in the cells homing to the lung capillaries, leading to improved lung function and quality of life. The study concluded that the therapeutic benefits were largely attributable to the paracrine effects and immune modulation facilitated by the localization of MSCs in the lung microenvironment.

To wrap this up on how stem cells actually create a therapeutic benefit, the capture of infused stem cells in the lung capillary beds plays a crucial role in their therapeutic effects for lung diseases such as COPD. This localization ensures that the paracrine signals, immune modulation, and regenerative capabilities of the stem cells are concentrated in the affected lung tissue.

As I have shown you now, evidence from both preclinical and clinical studies supports the importance of this mechanism in mediating positive outcomes. Were I to engage in future research, I would continue to explore the precise molecular and cellular interactions involved in this process to optimize stem cell therapies for lung diseases. It's this level of detailed research that will create a standardized treatment model.

Here's one key aspect of repeated value to this whole topic: if you infuse your own cells, you are not just getting a benefit to your lungs, you are getting a tremendous boost to your whole system. I have written extensively about longevity and stem cells for longevity.

The benefits to your whole system are substantial. Also, you can repeat this process of infusion over and over. To date, there has been no data that I'm aware of showing that infusions of your own cells are a bad, dangerous, or negative activity. It seems that all signs point to positive and health boosting outcomes.

Now that we've covered the specifics of how the actual stem cells interact with your lung tissue to produce benefits, let's explore a little more about the treatment process.

The Significance Of Stem Cells In COPD Treatment

I like to use an article to base a specific conversation on, so I have chosen this article to serve as the basis for a discussion on using your own autologous mesenchymal stem cells for a COPD treatment. "Autologous Infusion of Bone Marrow and Mesenchymal Stromal Cells in Patients with Chronic Obstructive Pulmonary Disease: Phase I Randomized Clinical Trial"

I'll summarize the article and make a few observations here for you. The article reports on a Phase I randomized clinical trial investigating the safety and potential efficacy of autologous infusion of bone marrow-derived mesenchymal stromal cells (MSCs) in patients with chronic obstructive pulmonary disease (COPD).

As we already know, COPD is a chronic and progressive lung disease characterized by airflow limitation, specifically the inability to exhale air. In medical school, we likened this situation to the difference between a normal balloon - when you blow air in it will naturally have a resistance tension that will help expire the air - whereas with COPD, you have damaged the tissues such that the elastic nature of the tissue will not retract and expire the air, which obviously significantly impairs quality of life through the inability to breathe normally. Current treatments primarily focus on symptom management, prompting the exploration of regenerative therapies like MSCs, which have anti-inflammatory and tissue repair properties.

The study enrolled COPD patients who were randomized to receive either an autologous infusion of bone marrow-derived MSCs or a placebo. I want to point out here that autologous mesenchymal stem cells can be harvested from either bone marrow or adipose fat tissue and there are numerous articles pointing out the similarities and benefits of each of these.

In the case of this article, bone marrow was harvested from the iliac crest of each patient, and MSCs were isolated, cultured, and expanded before being infused intravenously, which is the exact same model of therapy I have outlined above. For this article, they are tracking key outcomes, including safety, feasibility, and preliminary efficacy.

Here are the results:
The study found that the autologous infusion of MSCs was safe and well-tolerated by all patients. I want to re-emphasize that, well-tolerated by all patients, meaning it's a very safe treatment modality. There were no serious adverse events reported, and minor side effects were transient and manageable.

Usually when doing IVs you have normal issues with IV application like finding veins and bruising and such, but this is not reflective of the stem cell infusion itself, merely the application model. The feasibility of the procedure was confirmed, as MSCs were successfully isolated, cultured, and administered in all cases. Again, culture and expansion of stem cells is standard biotech procedure now.

Regarding efficacy, there were mixed results, but keep in mind that a single treatment event isn't necessarily the recommended therapy model. Chemo patients undergo multiple rounds of therapy for months. Many other treatment models for various illnesses and conditions require multiple courses of therapy and many months of duration.

This is why I'm such a proponent of owning your own stem cells for life in a manner that you'll never run out. Some patients showed modest improvements in lung function and quality of life, while others did not exhibit significant changes. This is common in general studies with small populations, some people just don't respond, but again, the severity of the condition of each patient also factors into this situation.

Side note: I know offices that screen their patients for a range of procedures so that they only accept patients that will have successful outcomes. They position this as being a candidate for the procedure. So this will artificially inflate their success rates because they are only accepting patients they are confident will have a positive outcome.

Imagine if I could conduct a trial that way, I could create amazing outcomes in all my studies! But real life is very different and not all things work for all people. In fact, having anything with a success rate over 50% is considered substantial in the medical field.

I know doctors who are trying to achieve 10-20% improvements in their patients' conditions. I also know patients who are willing to jump through a lot of hoops just to get that 10-20% improvement. Surgeons in hospitals are rated based on their successful outcomes as well, so they are very selective on who they will perform on and what scenarios they will perform on.

It's all about two things, making sure the patients actually have a chance to succeed in the procedure, and secondly, maintaining a positive reputation for that procedure in the public.

Nobody wants a surgeon with a 10% success rate, or a procedure with a 10% success rate, unless the alternative is 0% elsewhere. I like to point out again that autologous stem cell treatments are considered safe even if they are not producing an overwhelming success response for the condition being treated, and also there are a range of positive benefits across the body for doing these infusions of high dose stem cells.

So, all this said, just because the study doesn't show an overwhelming success rate doesn't mean that it's a negative outcome across the board for the patients that didn't respond. Not responding positively is also not responding negatively in this situation. At least it's not a drug with side effects, or a surgery with extreme risk of long-term malfunction and pain.

Tracking outcomes for COPD is pretty straightforward. Pulmonary function tests, such as Forced Expiratory Volume in one second (FEV1) and Forced Vital Capacity (FVC), showed variable responses.

Biomarkers of inflammation also showed inconsistent changes, with some patients experiencing reduced levels of inflammatory markers, suggesting a potential anti-inflammatory effect of the MSCs.

Quality of life is also one of the most important things to track. Did the patient feel better overall in the days/weeks/months after the treatment? It's important to pay attention to a range of possible benefits.

The authors discussed the implications of the findings, noting that while the safety and feasibility of autologous MSC infusion in COPD patients were established, the efficacy results were inconclusive, as is the safest way to report on something that is sure to get beat up by the entrenched medical authorities.

Stem cells for osteoarthritis and other MSK conditions were heavily fought against by the mainstream orthopedic doctors for years, but a few doctors just kept posting success after success until the mainstream docs just shut up a bit.

Note what you'll see is less negative commenting about it and more ignoring it by the mainstream docs. I expect the same with COPD for the next decade. No doctor of PhD is going to stake their career on this one study with a small sample size. They are going to state that more data is needed to know for sure if there's any benefit.

This Phase I trial demonstrated that autologous infusion of bone marrow-derived MSCs is a safe and feasible approach for COPD patients, with some indications of potential efficacy, which is the most we could hope for with an initial phase 1 study.

This study also serves as a foundation for future research aimed at refining stem cell therapy for COPD, ultimately aiming to improve the management and outcomes for patients with this challenging disease. Further studies with larger sample sizes and longer follow-up periods are essential to fully elucidate the therapeutic potential of MSCs in COPD.

Stem Cell Application Process

OK, so here is the big deal … the secret sauce … the secret ingredient of my secret ingredient soup (in case any of you have seen Kung-Fu Panda) for treatment of COPD: an IV infusion of your own stem cells that have been cultured and expanded.

It's actually a very simple process. I've talked to a lot of medical providers here in the US who are perfectly willing to do an IV of the patient's own cultured expanded stem cells. So, the process is fairly simple. After you have your own cells, a medical provider will perform the IV infusion, which is also a very simple process: a modest IV protocol where the cells are introduced over the course of a pretty short period of time, likely about an hour.

Some providers opt for different time frames and that's their call, but for the most part all the IV infusion scenarios are about the same.

It's that simple! So, why is it such a big deal? It's not an established treatment modality for mainstream medical, so it's just one of those things you have to expect will get push-back from mainstream doctors. However, like I said, I know a lot of providers who are perfectly happy to perform injections and IV of the patient's own cells.

It would be another story if the product they were injecting or infusing was a purchased birth tissue product, they would not be willing to do that, but if it's the patient's own cells they're likely to be fine with it.

So, that said, I go back to my original promotion of banking your own cells. You can bank your own stem cells and have stem cells for life, then you can do whatever you want with your cells the rest of your life. You'll never run out!

Conclusion And Solutions For COPD

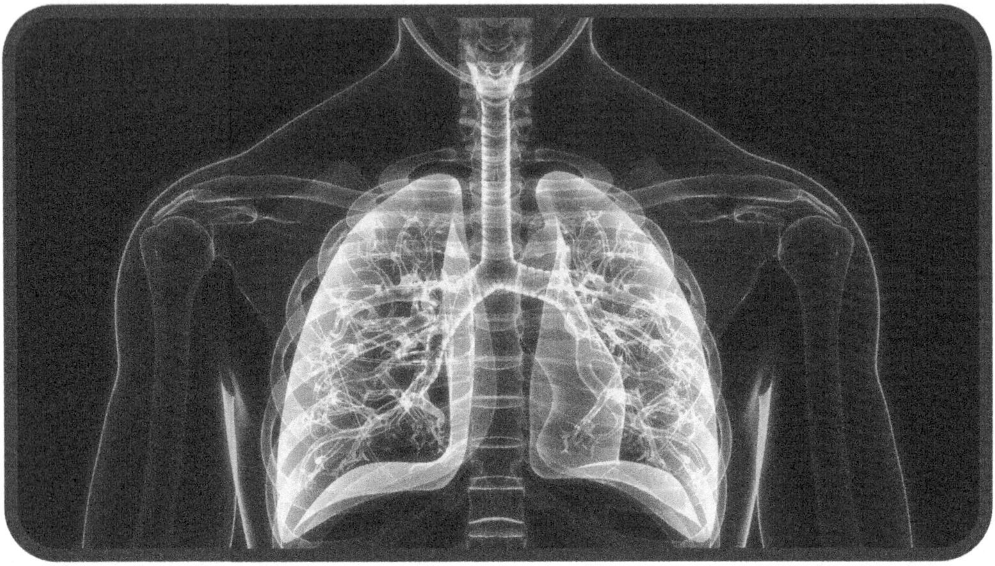

Stem cell therapy is probably one of, if not the only, realistically useful treatment for COPD out in the market today. I stand by the premise that your own cells are going to be the best option because you can grow and expand a lifetime supply of cells, and this is possible even if you are not "young" anymore.

Your stem cells can still be simulated and cultured and expanded. It's just a matter of getting it done. I recommend using Longevity Stem Cells, www.longevitystemcells.com as the lab service that can culture and expand your adipose stem cells into high dose stem cells. If you have questions about this process or this company, just reach out to me and I'll help.

Regarding traveling overseas, you don't need to!!! If you have a doctor selling you on the idea of traveling overseas to a Central American nation to get a very expensive stem cell treatment, you definitely need to talk to me first. You can get this all done here in the US now and for much less than what you're seeing in these expensive travel trips.

Seriously, reach out to me first before you pay for one of those packages, I don't care how nice or convincing your doctor or chiropractor is, if they are referring you to an overseas clinic they are likely making money on that transaction and that's part of why it's so expensive.

- Caveat on Autologous Stem Cells: If you are not in a state of health or condition where you could safely engage in an adipose collection procedure to have your cells cultured and expanded, and you believe you are in need of cultured/expanded donor cells, allogeneic stem cells, then yes, you would need to travel to obtain this treatment, as most doctors in the US are unwilling to engage in cultured expanded donor cell therapy.

  The international stem cell market is very active in this category. I can also recommend centers that are reputable so you don't end up in a shady place with stem cells you can't track or document.

By now you have learned quite a bit more than most people know or understand about stem cells and stem cell therapy options inside and outside the US medical market.

Also, I hope you know more about some of the other excellent non-stem cell options available here in the US that are still excellent starting points for anyone suffering from a condition where stem cells would be a great option.

Your options in the US are tremendous, so I don't want anyone to think that they can't get some of the best treatments in the world here in the US. The expanded cell therapy market outside the US is much more expensive and difficult to navigate, so I don't like telling people to just go get the latest and greatest from anywhere in the world.

I want to make sure those options are vetted, so people asking me are going to the right places. Always reach out to me on my personal site to ask about where to go for whatever you're looking for.

My experience in the biotech field and in owning and operating multiple biotech labs and medical practices and various other lab companies has helped me appreciate the complexity of this new era of stem cell therapy. I'm confident in the future of medicine and what we can accomplish.

It may be scary to some, but after years of seeing doctors and patients warm up to the new therapy options, and seeing the results, I'm confident that a new wave of acceptance in stem cell therapy will continue to trigger new advancements in the field.

I maintain connections across the nation and the world on regenerative medicine to keep my finger on the pulse of what's going on and what is being developed.

If you are uncertain about what you're being told, or what you're reading, promises of cures and treatments being presented, or even the price of the therapy being offered, reach out to me and I'll help guide you.

I can dig into just about any marketing pitch from any practice and see what they are actually offering. Most of them are repackaging the same things I've seen a thousand times!

I may not be able to advocate for you directly, but I can help guide you on your journey. At the very least I can send you to people who I know will take care of you properly and not simply recite some marketing material to you or promise you the world and a lifetime of health and happiness for a swipe of your credit card. Let's work together to make regenerative medicine the field it's meant to be and advocate for the good and eliminate the bad. We can do it together!

I look forward to seeing, talking, and connecting with you directly on my personal site and my business sites willbozeman.com, www.relatyv.com, www.longevitystemcells.com, and www.regenenesthetics.com, as well as any of my social media accounts:

- Twitter: @WBozeman70246
- Facebook: @WillBozeman
- LinkedIn: @will-bozeman
- Instagram: @willbozemanceo

Thank you so much for reading this book and taking the leap to learn more about this new era of medicine. My last request is that after you have read this book and you've connected with me to guide you on where to go for treatment, give this book to someone else who needs it and help them find what they are looking for!

Every little thing we can do for one of us will help all of us!

Made in the USA
Monee, IL
04 November 2026

67381197R00075